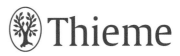

Hand Trauma:
Illustrated Surgical Guide of Core Procedures

Dariush Nikkhah, BM, MSc, MRCS (Eng)
Plastic Surgery Registrar
Barts and The Royal London NHS Trust
London, UK

389 illustrations

Thieme
Stuttgart • New York • Delhi • Rio de Janeiro

Library of Congress Cataloging-in-Publication Data

Names: Nikkhah, Dariush, author.

Title: Hand trauma : illustrated surgical guide of core procedures / Dariush Nikkhah.

Description: Stuttgart ; New York : Thieme, [2018] | Includes bibliographical references and index.

Identifiers: LCCN 2017029140 (print) | LCCN 2017029568 (ebook) | ISBN 9783132414266 | ISBN 9783132414365 (eISBN)

Subjects: | MESH: Hand Injuries–surgery | Hand Injuries–rehabilitation | Hand–surgery | Surgical Flaps

Classification: LCC RD559 (ebook) | LCC RD559 (print) | NLM WE 832 | DDC 617.5/75044–dc23

LC record available at https://lccn.loc.gov/2017029140

© 2018 by Georg Thieme Verlag KG

Thieme Publishers Stuttgart
Rüdigerstrasse 14, 70469 Stuttgart, Germany
+49 [0]711 8931 421, customerservice@thieme.de

Thieme Publishers New York
333 Seventh Avenue, New York, NY 10001 USA
+1 800 782 3488, customerservice@thieme.com

Thieme Publishers Delhi
A-12, Second Floor, Sector-2, Noida-201301
Uttar Pradesh, India
+91 120 45 566 00, customerservice@thieme.in

Thieme Publishers Rio, Thieme Publicações Ltda.
Edifício Rodolpho de Paoli, 25º andar
Av. Nilo Peçanha, 50 – Sala 2508,
Rio de Janeiro 20020-906 Brasil
Tel: +55 21 3172-2297 / +55 21 3172-1896

Cover design: Thieme Publishing Group
Typesetting by Thomson Digital, India

Printed in India by Replika Press Pvt. Ltd.   5 4 3 2 1

ISBN 978-3-13-241426-6

Also available as an e-book:
eISBN 978-3-13-241436-5

Important Note: Medicine is an ever-changing science undergoing continual development. Research and clinical experience are continually expanding our knowledge, in particular our knowledge of proper treatment and drug therapy. Insofar as this book mentions any dosage or application, readers may rest assured that the authors, editors, and publishers have made every effort to ensure that such references are in accordance with **the state of knowledge at the time of production of the book.**

Nevertheless, this does not involve, imply, or express any guarantee or responsibility on the part of the publishers with respect of any dosage instructions and forms of application stated in the book. **Every user is requested to examine carefully** the manufacturer's leaflets accompanying each drug and to check, if necessary in consultation with a physician or specialist, whether the dosage schedules mentioned therein or the contraindications stated by the manufacturer differ from the statements made in the present book. Such examination is particularly important with drugs that are either rarely used or have been newly released on the market. Every dosage schedule or every form of application used is entirely at the user's risk and responsibility. The authors and publishers request every user to report to the publishers any discrepancies or inaccuracies noticed.

Some of the product names, patents, and registered designs referred to in this book are in fact registered trademarks or proprietary names, even though specific reference to this fact is not always made in the text. Therefore, the appearance of a name without a designation as proprietary is not to be construed as a representation by the publisher that it is in the public domain.

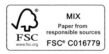

This book would not have been possible without all the great teachers and mentors I have had in my training.

I must thank my father and mother, who have given me all the opportunities throughout my life.

I must also thank my dearest wife, Mahdis, who supported me through the writing of this book.

This book is also in memory of my grandparents, whose footsteps I follow.

Contents

Contents

Foreword

The author should be congratulated for turning a great idea into a very readable, practical, and useful textbook on surgical techniques for the management of hand injuries. I can think of no other textbook that provides this sort of clear guidance for many of the commonly used basic surgical techniques (plus many useful tips and tricks) that will help training surgeons safely and effectively manage day-to-day hand trauma. The text has deliberately been kept light; readers will find that the images in the book provide a very clear explanation of the techniques that are being described, whether it is for fracture management or tendon repair. I honestly think that this will be an invaluable source of information to junior orthopaedic and plastic surgery trainees learning about and applying basic surgical techniques for the management of hand trauma. Details of useful references will allow readers who wish to dig a little deeper to get further information on the subjects that are covered in each of the chapters of the book. I predict that this will be a valuable addition to the libraries of young surgeons involved in treating patients with upper limb injuries.

Mark Pickford, MD, FRCS (Plast)
Consultant Plastic and Hand Surgeon
Queen Victoria Hospital
East Grinstead
Sussex, UK

Preface

Treatment of hand trauma is an art and it requires mastery of several different disciplines. The diversity of this surgical field includes topics ranging from microsurgery of vessels less than 1 mm in diameter, to osteosynthesis, and flap coverage of traumatic defects. It requires creativity and is constantly being innovated. This book cannot cover all relevant procedures, but it aims to help the trainee understand core principles.

For a trainee in surgery, it is useful to have a resource that summarizes and explains the fundamental steps in an operation. All operations can be viewed as sequences of steps and this is particularly the case in hand surgery. As a trainee, I had the opportunity to learn technical tips and tricks that I want to share. These may prove useful for the management of patients. The majority of the cases explained in the book are patients I have operated upon in my training. *This is a book "for the registrars, by the registrars."*

The available literature has only a few books that use sequential annotated pictures to illustrate basic hand trauma procedures. I hope this book will be a useful resource to the on-call surgeon seeking accessible advice and help, as the figures and commentary can be used as an aide-mémoire in challenging cases. The book is not supposed to be an exhaustive compendium of different surgical techniques in hand trauma, nor does it claim that the techniques illustrated in it are superior to others described elsewhere. Its objective is simply to describe principles and technical tips that I have found useful and effective in my training.

To quote Wayne Morrison: *"Emergency surgery is learnt in the trenches."*[1] This stepwise guide will hopefully aid trainees safely find their way through no man's land.

Dariush Nikkhah, BM, MSc, MRCS (Eng)
Plastic Surgery Registrar
Barts and The Royal London NHS trust
London, UK

[1] Morrison WA, McCombe D. Digital replantation. Hand Clin. 2007; 23(1):1–12

Acknowledgments

I would like to express my deepest gratitude to my trainers and mentors: Mark Pickford, Norbert Kang, TC Teo, Neil Toft, Bran Sivakumar, Baljit Dheansa, Martin Jones, Wikus De Jager, and Mohammed Shibu. All of them trained me and pushed me as a Junior Registrar.

I must also thank Guj Pahal for several images that he provided.

I would also like to convey special thanks to my father, Dr Jamshid Nikkhah, who supported me through all my training and is still a constant source of advice.

Finally, I would also like to thank Stephan Konnry of Thieme Medical Publishers for his immediate, enthusiastic response to this book. Furthermore, I must thank my editor, Sapna Rastogi, for her tireless editing of the final version of the book.

Contributors

Mo Akhavani, FRCS (Plast)
Consultant Plastic Surgeon
Royal Free Hospital
Hampstead, UK

Nikki Burr, MSc
Consultant Hand Therapist
Mount Vernon and Royal Free Hospitals
London, UK

Wojciech Konczalik, BSc, MRCS
Registrar in Plastic Surgery
Royal Free Hospital
Hampstead, UK

Robert Pearl, MD, FRCS (Plast)
Consultant Plastic Surgeon
Queen Victoria Hospital
East Grinstead
Sussex, UK

Jeremy Prout, FRCA
Consultant Anaesthetist
Royal Free Hospital
London, UK

Jeremy Rodrigues, MSc, MRCS, PhD
Registrar in Plastic Surgery
University of Oxford
Oxford, UK

Amir H. Sadr, MSc, MRCS
Registrar in Plastic Surgery
Royal Free Hospital
London, UK

Stamatis Sapzountzis, MD
Consultant Plastic Surgeon
St Luke's Hospital
Thessaloniki, Greece

Roshan Vijayan, MSc, MRCS
Registrar in Plastic Surgery
Barts and The Royal London NHS Trust
London, UK

1 Assessment

Dariush Nikkhah, Jeremy Rodrigues

Keywords: flexor tendon, extensor tendon, static two-point discrimination, tenodesis, central slip

The primary assessment of the hand injury is like good detective work. It can enable the surgeon to exactly predict which structures may be damaged and need to be identified during the surgery.

1.1 History

History should begin with the occupation and hand dominance of the patient. The mechanism of injury is important and can give clues before surgery is

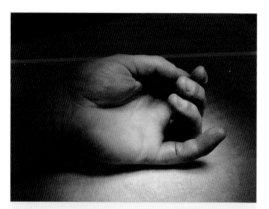

Fig. 1.1 The hand demonstrating abnormal cascade after zone 2 flexor tendon laceration to the little finger.

undertaken, for example, knowledge of the type of saw blade can forewarn the surgeon of possible segmental defects in structures. Powered saws tend to result in segmental defects. Relevant past medical history helps to determine the patient's anesthetic risk.

1.2 Examination

1.2.1 Look

Inspect the cascade of the digits of the hand and identify any obvious irregularity (► Fig. 1.1, ► Fig. 1.2, ► Fig. 1.3). All fingertips should naturally tend to flex toward the scaphoid tubercle (► Fig. 1.4). Always compare both hands. Assess for wound vascularity by assessing capillary refill at the pulp of the injured digits.

Rotational deformities resulting in scissoring of digits should be documented (► Fig. 1.5, ► Fig. 1.6).

In ► Fig. 1.2 and ► Fig. 1.3, the patient has suffered a knife laceration that has resulted in the division of his or her flexor tendons. Therefore, the normal cascade has been disrupted.

1.2.2 Feel

Sensation can be tested with static two-point discrimination (S2PD) (► Fig. 1.7, ► Fig. 1.8). Suspect sensory nerve injury if S2PD is greater than 5 mm or the patient has lost the ability to discriminate

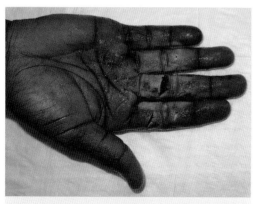

Fig. 1.2 Knife laceration involving index, middle, and ring fingers.

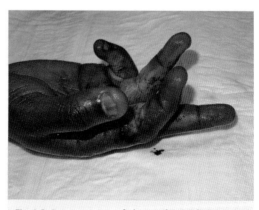

Fig. 1.3 Demonstration of abnormal cascade.

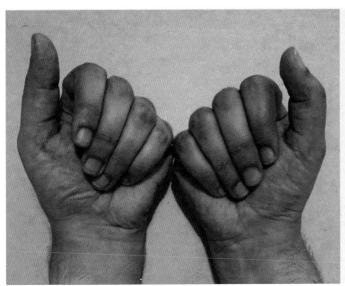

Fig. 1.4 Demonstration of no rotational deformities or scissoring in the normal hand.

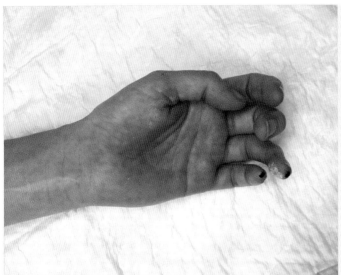

Fig. 1.5 Proximal phalanx fracture of the ring finger resulting in scissoring.

between one versus two pinpoints. It is important to note that some patients struggle to do this on normal digits and comparison must be made on the uninjured side.

In young children, the tactile adherence test can be used to assess the digital nerve. When gently brushed along a normal digit, a plastic pen will *drag* due to the normal perspiration. In denervated areas, sweating gets stopped, and this drag is lost; the pen slides with less friction.

Sensory loss in the median, ulnar, and radial nerve distributions should be mapped and documented.

1.2.3 Move

Assess whether the patient can make a full fist actively or if there are any issues with their range of motion or rotation. Test for joint instability and laxity after a possible joint dislocation.

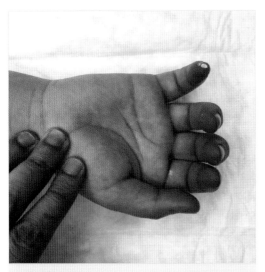

Fig. 1.6 Abnormal digital cascade in a child with a Salter-Harris II proximal phalanx fracture of the little finger.

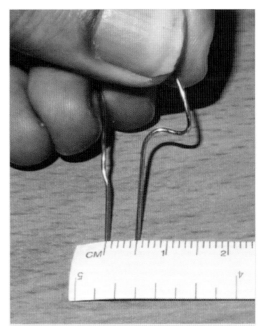

Fig. 1.7 One can calibrate a two-point discriminator with a paperclip and ruler.

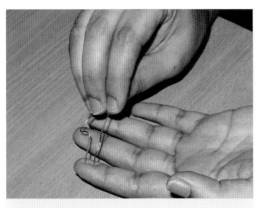

Fig. 1.8 Testing S2PD on fingertips using calibrated paper clip set at 5 mm.

Examine the power of the extensors and flexors individually. If the patient has active movement, but there is pain against resistance, this could be suggestive of a partial tendon injury.

Extensor pollicis longus (EPL) is tested by placing the hand flat on the table and asking the patient to raise the thumb up into the air. This movement is called retropulsion (▶ Fig. 1.9).

Test the flexor digitorum superficialis (FDS) tendon by holding other fingers extended (this prevents the flexor digitorum profundus [FDP] action) while the affected finger is actively flexed by the patient (▶ Fig. 1.10). FDP is tested by the patient actively flexing the distal interphalangeal joint (DIPJ) (▶ Fig. 1.11).

The central slip (zone 3) of the extensor tendon can be examined by performing the central slip tenodesis test. This involves passively flexing the wrist fully, and then the metacarpophalangeal joint (MCPJ) by gently applying pressure to the dorsum of the proximal phalanx. If there is disruption of the central slip, there will be a persistent extensor lag at the proximal interphalangeal joint (PIPJ). In contrast, with an intact central slip, there will be passive extension of the PIPJ as the MCPJ is flexed (▶ Fig. 1.12).

The tenodesis effect can also be used to assess for flexor injury. Passive wrist flexion and extension of a relaxed hand assess tenodesis. If the flexor tendons are intact, wrist extension causes passive flexion of the digits. However, if the digits do not flex, this is suggestive of flexor tendon injury (▶ Fig. 1.13a,b).

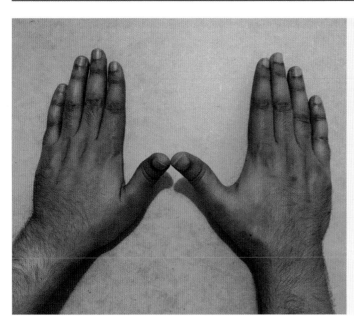

Fig. 1.9 EPL retropulsion test, place palm flat on table and move thumb to the ceiling.

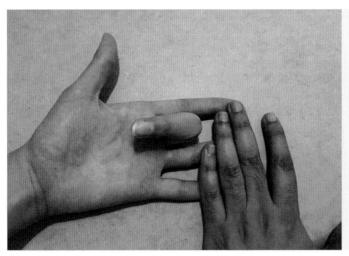

Fig. 1.10 Testing middle finger FDS.

Thumb palmar abduction can be performed to check the motor function of the median nerve (▶ Fig. 1.14) and adduction and abduction of the digits can be tested for assessment of the ulnar nerve motor function (▶ Fig. 1.15a,b).

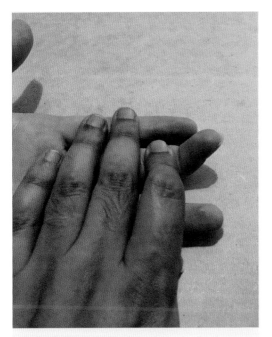

Fig. 1.11 Testing middle finger FDP.

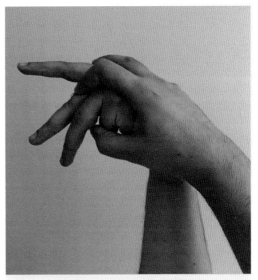

Fig. 1.12 Central slip tenodesis test of right middle finger demonstrating intact central slip due to passive extension of PIPJ.

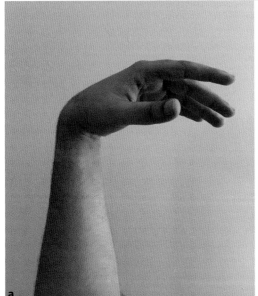

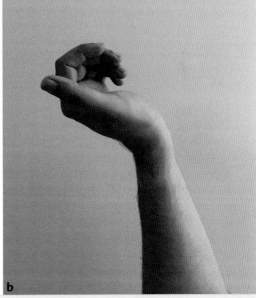

a **b**

Fig. 1.13 Tenodesis test. (a) Passive wrist flexion. (b) Passive wrist extension.

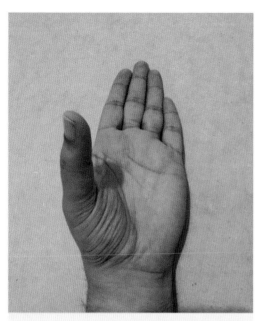

Fig. 1.14 Thumb abduction assessing the abductor pollicis brevis.

1.3 Investigations

Investigations can include radiographs, which should be taken with three views. Blood tests such as C-reactive protein (CRP) and erythrocyte sedimentation rate (ESR) can be done in cases of acute infection as a baseline test. Further tests such as oxygen saturation probe can be used to determine vascularity (▶ Fig. 1.16).

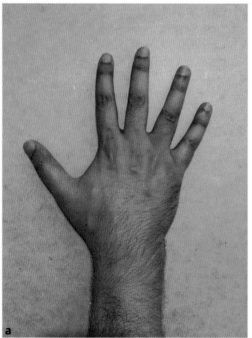
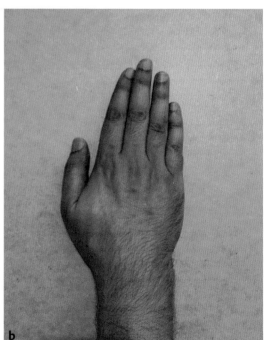

Fig. 1.15 (a) Finger abduction. **(b)** Finger adduction.

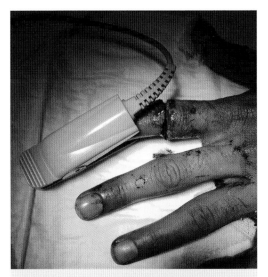

Fig. 1.16 Use of a pulse oximeter in a circumferential laceration with questionable capillary refill. This technique is useful in triage of hand trauma patients where vascularity is uncertain clinically and provides a reliable objective measure.

Selected Readings

Finnell JT, Knopp R, Johnson P, Holland PC, Schubert W. A calibrated paper clip is a reliable measure of two-point discrimination. Acad Emerg Med. 2004; 11(6):710–714

The authors compared two different instruments for assessing digital two-point discrimination. The authors found that a calibrated bent paper clip performed as well as the Disk-Criminator.

Harrison SH. The tactile adherence test estimating loss of sensation after nerve injury. Hand. 1974; 6(2):148–149

Original description of the most commonly used tests in young or uncooperative patients—the ballpoint pen test. The ballpoint pen is drawn across the surface of the skin, and loss of adherence can be seen in areas of anhidrosis. Sweat production is dependent on sympathetic fibers, which are very resistant to mechanical trauma, which is why damage to these fibers points toward a significant nerve injury.

Louis DS, Greene TL, Jacobson KE, Rasmussen C, Kolowich P, Goldstein SA. Evaluation of normal values for stationary and moving two-point discrimination in the hand. J Hand Surg Am. 1984; 9 (4):552–555

Reports a study of stationary and moving two-point discrimination in a normal population stratified by age and sex. Moving two-point values were found to be of lower magnitude than stationary two-point values in all areas of the hand. Median nerve innervated areas had more accurate two-point discrimination than ulnar nerve innervated regions. Women had more accurate two-point discrimination than men in all areas of the hand. Absolute values were found to be examiner dependent. However, the findings were based on the pooled data of examiners.

Smith PJ, Ross DA. The central slip tenodesis test for early diagnosis of potential boutonnière deformities. J Hand Surg [Br]. 1994; 19 (1):88–90

The authors describe a simple, noninvasive test for assessment of central slip disruption. This test avoids those many problems that are encountered in other tests due to pain.

Tarabadkar N, Iorio ML, Gundle K, Friedrich JB. The use of pulse oximetry for objective quantification of vascular injuries in the hand. Plast Reconstr Surg. 2015; 136(6):1227–1233

Evaluation of the efficacy of pulse oximetry as a proxy for digital perfusion in penetrating injuries of the fingers. Twenty patients with a total of 49 digital lacerations were included in the study. Pulse oximetry readings were recorded prior to surgical exploration. A statistically significant difference was found between the digits that had vascular injury necessitating repair versus those that did not. Data suggest that an arterial oxygen saturation (SaO_2) of 97% or above is associated with vascular injury being highly improbable and all digits in the study with SaO_2 84% or lower had vascular injury needing repair.

2 Operative Preparation

Dariush Nikkhah, Jeremy Rodrigues

Keywords: tourniquet, theater lighting, wide-awake hand surgery

2.1 Tourniquet Application

Appropriate placement of a tourniquet is essential and is usually performed before skin preparation, unless a sterile tourniquet is being used. Two loops of wool or similar should be wrapped around the arm before tourniquet application. More than two loops may result in a loss of pressure applied to the arm (▶ Fig. 2.1, ▶ Fig. 2.2). Furthermore, adhesive

tape should be placed around the tourniquet (▶ Fig. 2.3). This prevents any prep solution leaking under the tourniquet which would risk causing a chemical burn. Tourniquet burns are indefensible.

2.2 Theater Draping and Lighting

The hand is prepared with an antiseptic solution. If the arm is paralyzed or the patient is under general anesthetic, an unscrubbed member of the theater team holds the arm up to facilitate the skin preparation (▶ Fig. 2.4).

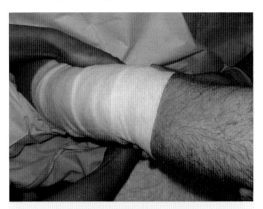

Fig. 2.1 Applying roll of soft band padding.

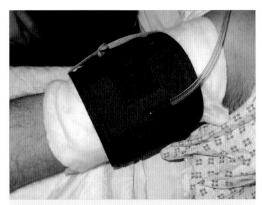

Fig. 2.2 Application of tourniquet over padding.

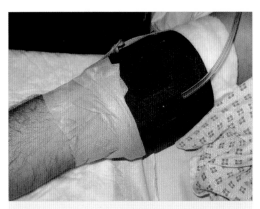

Fig. 2.3 Ensure adhesive tape prevents the prep from going underneath the tourniquet.

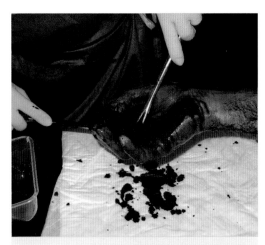

Fig. 2.4 The assistant holds the arm while the scrub nurse preps the arm with Betadine using both sponges.

In some instances, if the hand is contaminated and embedded with particulate matter, a prescrub is necessary with a disposable nailbrush. The hand is then passed through an aperture drape and the primary surgeon should sit on the ulnar side of the hand (▶ Fig. 2.5, ▶ Fig. 2.6). Two theater lights should be positioned in the direction of the patient's hand with the surgeon sitting in between the two lights (▶ Fig. 2.7).

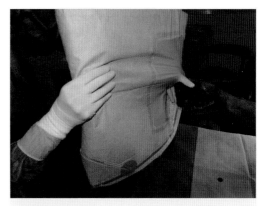

Fig. 2.5 Pass the hand through aperture drape.

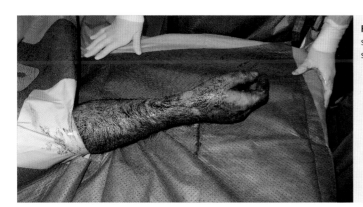

Fig. 2.6 The primary surgeon should sit on the ulnar side of the hand once sterile drapes have been placed.

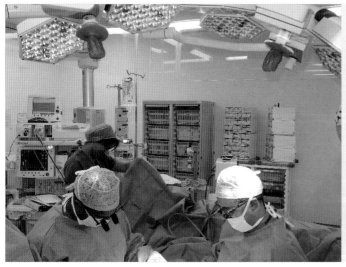

Fig. 2.7 Two theater lights positioned in the direction of the patient's hand with the surgeon sitting in between the two lights for optimal lighting.

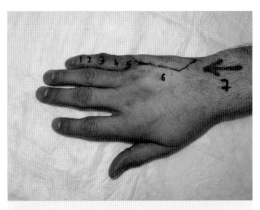

Fig. 2.8 Wide-awake hand surgery after anesthetic infiltration of 0.5% bupivacaine with 1 in 200,000 adrenaline. The extensor zones are labeled in the illustration.

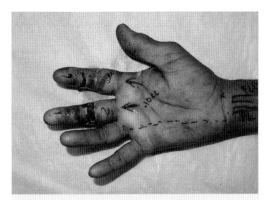

Fig. 2.9 Wide-awake exploration of index and middle fingers after flexor zone 2 tendon injuries. About 10 mL tumescent of 1% lignocaine with 1:100,000 adrenaline is administered into the palm. Note the white area of vasoconstriction after 30 minutes in the illustration. Further injection of 2 mL is given in the subcutaneous fat of the proximal phalanx and middle phalanx, respectively. The injection in the digit is given in the midline between the digital nerves. A final 1 mL injection is given in the pulp.

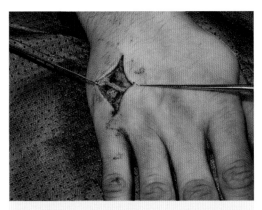

Fig. 2.10 Case in ▶ Fig. 2.8 demonstrating minimal bleeding after exploration at 30 minutes.

2.3 Surgery without a Tourniquet

It is also possible to operate without a tourniquet using local anesthetic and adrenaline tumescent technique as described by Lalonde (▶ Fig. 2.8, ▶ Fig. 2.9). This approach achieves a chemical tourniquet. This is particularly useful in cases of tendon transfer and tendon repair, as active movement by the patient is preserved and can be used to optimize tendon tension. Ideally, 30 minutes is allowed to elapse between infiltration and incision. Although this technique does not always achieve a bloodless field, it eliminates problems

such as tourniquet pain and the need for sedation (▶ Fig. 2.10).

Selected Readings

Chiang YC, Lin TS, Yeh MC. Povidone-iodine-related burn under the tourniquet of a child—a case report and literature review. J Plast Reconstr Aesthet Surg. 2011; 64(3):412–415

A report of two cases of chemical burns following 10% povidone-iodine solution getting into the padding of tourniquet during lower limb surgery. The mechanism of the burn results from a combination of skin maceration, increased pressure from the tourniquet, and direct irritation from the antiseptic solution. Chronic ulceration, scar hypertrophy, and hypersensitivity are possible complications. Application of an adhesive plaster to serve as a mechanical barrier can eliminate this risk.

Lalonde D, Martin A. Tumescent local anesthesia for hand surgery: improved results, cost effectiveness, and wide-awake patient satisfaction. Arch Plast Surg. 2014; 41(4):312–316

Review of wide-awake local anesthesia no tourniquet (WALANT) hand surgery. Evidence supports use of adrenaline solutions in digits with no reports of digital ischemia in the last 50 years. The technique is also cost-effective, as there is no need for preoperative testing as well as anesthetic and recovery room staff. Patient satisfaction is high as they are able to communicate freely with the surgeon during the operation. It also enables the surgeon to ask the patient to move his or her hand during the operation, which proves useful when testing tendon repairs or tensioning tendon transfers.

Lalonde DH, Wong A. Dosage of local anesthesia in wide awake hand surgery. J Hand Surg Am. 2013; 38(10):2025–2028

Article describes principles of anesthetic administration in wide-awake hand surgery. Lignocaine with adrenaline is injected subcutaneously via a 27-gauge needle in the area where the surgery will take place 30 minutes before the procedure. To minimize discomfort, 2 mL of anesthetic is injected immediately deep to dermis and this is allowed to take effect prior to further needle advancement. As the needle is passed forward, the solution is introduced 1 cm from the edge of the numb area to avoid injection pressure pain. Further needle insertion sites should always be sited in previously anesthetized areas.

Rajpura A, Somanchi BV, Muir LT. The effect of tourniquet padding on the efficiency of tourniquets of the upper limb. J Bone Joint Surg Br. 2007; 89(4):532–534

Study evaluating the effect of padding on the effectiveness of tourniquets in upper limb surgery. Two commonly used types of padding were compared (Velband and Cellona) and a varying number of layers were applied. A total of three pressure transducers were placed underneath the padding and the tourniquet was inflated to 220 mm Hg. Increasing number of layers reduced the pressure transmitted from the tourniquet, and this effect was found to be more pronounced with increasing arm circumference. Authors recommend that no more than two layers of padding should be used, as more layers will result in significant reductions in transmitted pressures.

3 Incisions

Dariush Nikkhah

Keywords: Bruner flap, midlateral incision

3.1 Bruner Flap

The Bruner flap is a commonly performed access incision and the modified version involves a broader

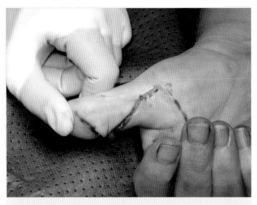

Fig. 3.1 Broad Bruner flaps in an adult.

flap. The most common mistake in flap design is making the angle of the flap too acute and therefore risking necrosis of the flap tip. This can be avoided if the flaps are designed with broad curved tips (▶ Fig. 3.1). This is a critical step because if the flaps fail over a tendon repair, the patient could develop tendon exposure and subsequent infection.

In children, Bruner-type incisions should be used as midlateral incisions which can often migrate volarly with growth, resulting in flexion contractures (▶ Fig. 3.2).

3.2 Midlateral Incision

The patient in ▶ Fig. 3.3 has sustained flexor zone 2 tendon injuries to four fingers secondary to a knife laceration. As his hand was clenched at the time, the level of tendon injury differs from the level of skin injury when the hand is relaxed. Midlateral access was performed in all digits within 45 minutes, before repairs were performed (▶ Fig. 3.3). The incision is marked by flexing the

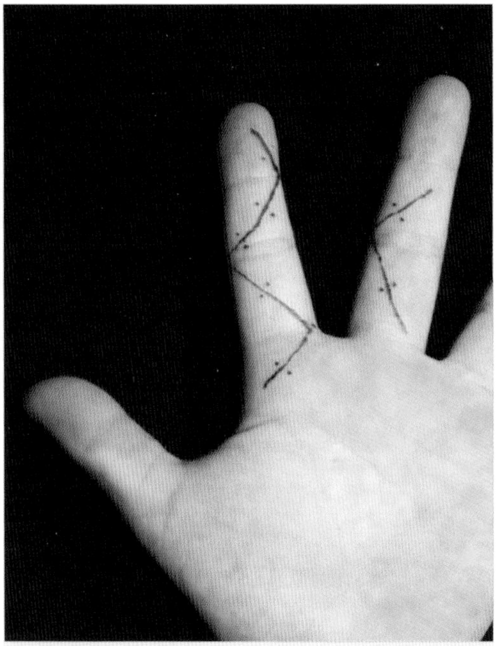

Fig. 3.2 Broad Bruner flaps in children, reaching midlateral lines. (This image is provided courtesy of Bran Sivakumar.)

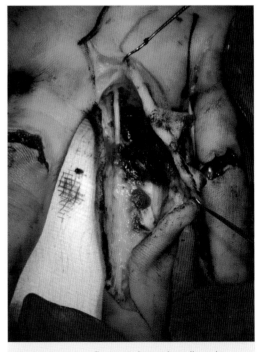

Fig. 3.3 Access to flexor tendon with midlateral approach.

digit and marking a point at the end of the flexion crease at each joint (▶ Fig. 3.4).

The midlateral approach is preferred by some hand surgeons as it avoids problems with flap necrosis as one broad flap is raised. It also avoids additional scarring over the site of the flexor tendon repair.

In the midlateral approach, the dorsal branch of the digital nerve is at risk and should be protected.

3.3 Extensor Access

The extensor tendons can be accessed via curvilinear incisions over the digits and dorsum of the hand. Again, the same principles apply with broad flaps and sufficient exposure so that tenorrhaphy can be undertaken without difficulty (▶ Fig. 3.5, ▶ Fig. 3.6, ▶ Fig. 3.7, ▶ Fig. 3.8).

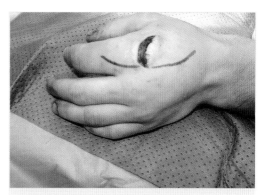

Fig. 3.5 Curvilinear extension markings for glass laceration over extensor zone 5.

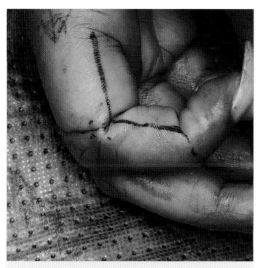

Fig. 3.4 Marking a point at the end of the flexion crease of each joint for midlateral access.

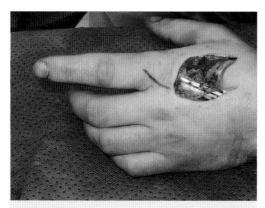

Fig. 3.6 Repair of the extensor digitorum communis (EDC) tendon over zone 5.

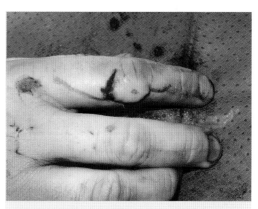

Fig. 3.7 Proximal interphalangeal joint (PIPJ) extensor zone 3 access. Note broad curvilinear flaps planned.

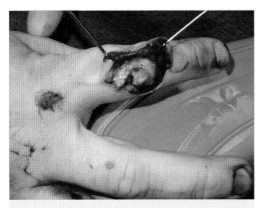

Fig. 3.8 Exposure demonstrates 90% division of central slip.

Selected Readings

Bruner JM. Surgical exposure of flexor tendons in the hand. Ann R Coll Surg Engl. 1973; 53(2):84–94

Paper written by Julian Bruner summarizing his 25-year experience of flexor tendon repair and incisions in hand surgery. Describes the principles underlying the extension of preexisting lacerations in the hand and wrist region. A discussion of the technical aspects of zig-zag and Bunnell's midlateral incision is present.

Tubiana R, Gilbert A, Masquelet AC, Dorn L. An Atlas of Surgical Techniques of the Hand and Wrist. 1st ed. London, UK: Martin Dunitz; 1999

Surgical atlas of operations of the hand and wrist. It is a step-by-step guide encompassing both elective and emergency procedures with over 800 illustrations. The technique, anatomy, common mistakes, and alternative options for common hand operations are described. In its description of designing skin incisions, it recommends that each incision in the palm is approximately 2.5 cm in length and that the flap tips have an angle greater than 30 degrees, with no incision crossing perpendicular to a joint crease.

4 Anesthesia in Hand Surgery

Dariush Nikkhah, Wojciech Konczalik, Jeremy Prout

Keywords: brachial plexus anesthesia, digital nerve block, wrist block

Many procedures in hand trauma can be performed under local anesthetic and patients can be managed in a day case setting. Some surgeons advocate surgery without a tourniquet using local anesthetic and adrenaline; however, this is not always suitable in complex multidigit injuries.

Wrist block can provide good local anesthesia; however, many patients suffer from significant tourniquet pain when this is performed without general anesthetic.

Most departments now use regional anesthesia in the form of brachial plexus anesthesia to provide effective postoperative pain relief. This avoids a general anesthetic (GA) and can be an efficient method of anesthesia if there is a block room available in the hand unit.

4.1 Wrist Block

The wrist block involves blocking the median nerve, ulnar nerve, and the sensory branch of the radial nerve. Key surface landmarks are identified for accurate placement of the injections (▶ Fig. 4.1). The aim is to inject close to but not directly into the nerves. Always withdraw on the plunger prior to infiltration to reduce the risk of intravascular injection.

The median nerve can be found deep into the palmaris longus tendon and the ulnar nerve runs radial and deep to the flexor carpi ulnaris tendon (▶ Fig. 4.2, ▶ Fig. 4.3). The dorsal branch of the ulnar nerve and palmar cutaneous branch of the median nerve often require separate injections (▶ Fig. 4.4). Finally, the sensory branch of the radial nerve should be blocked over the first extensor compartment (▶ Fig. 4.5).

Be careful to avoid an intraneural injection; sharp painful paresthesia in the distribution of a nerve territory upon siting the needle or during infiltration is suggestive of an intraneural injection. In such a case, the infiltration should be stopped and the needle should be repositioned prior to continuing.

4.2 Digital Nerve Block

Injections in the palm can be very painful; therefore, a dorsal approach to anesthetizing the digits may be considered preferable. Two injections are made to block the radial and ulnar digital nerves, after aspirating on the syringe plunger to avoid intravascular injection (▶ Fig. 4.6a,b). A final injection is made over the dorsum of the digit to block small dorsal nerves (▶ Fig. 4.6c). Alternatively, the flexor sheath can be blocked.

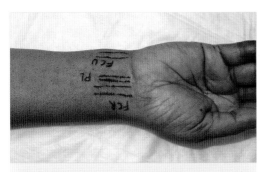

Fig. 4.1 Key landmarks to palpate before wrist block: palmaris longus and flexor carpi radialis (FCR) and flexor carpi ulnaris (FCU). The palmaris longus (PL) can be identified by thumb opposition and wrist flexion but is not always present in all patients.

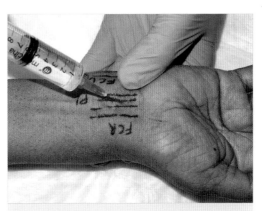

Fig. 4.2 Median nerve block: to block the median nerve one should aim between the palmaris longus (PL) and flexor carpi radialis (FCR).

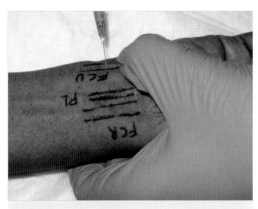

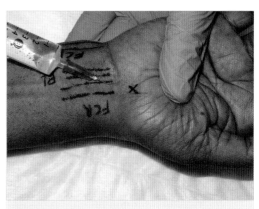

Fig. 4.3 Ulnar nerve block: the needle enters the skin ulnar and dorsal to the FCU heading radially and volarly toward the ulnar nerve (which lies radial to FCU). One should aspirate before injection to avoid injection into the ulnar artery.

Fig. 4.4 Injection of palmar cutaneous branch of median nerve marked with an "X."

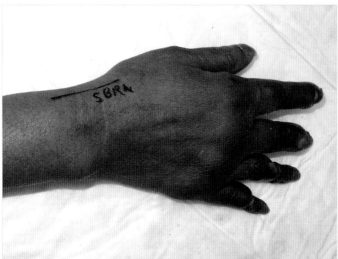

Fig. 4.5 Sensory branch of radial nerve over the first extensor compartment: local anesthetic fanned across this region provides anesthesia.

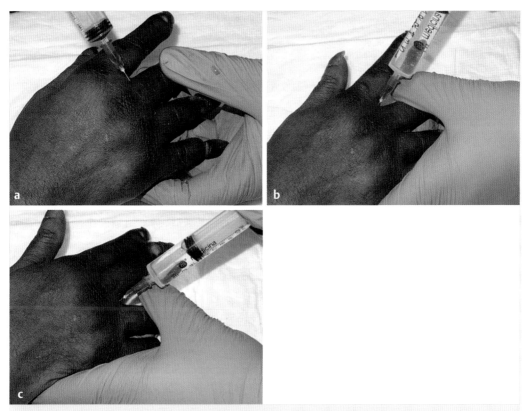

Fig. 4.6 (a–c) Digital nerve block, performed with three injections over dorsal aspect of digit. This is less painful than performing the injections through the palm. One must ensure to withdraw on the plungers so that local anesthetic is not injected into the digital arteries.

4.3 Brachial Plexus Block

Brachial plexus anesthesia can be administered as a single bolus or an infusion. The latter may also be continued postoperatively to encourage early rehabilitation. In selected cases, it can obviate the need for a GA and if used in combination with GA, it reduces complications such as headaches, nausea, and vomiting. There are several approaches to brachial plexus anesthesia: axillary, interscalene, supraclavicular, and infraclavicular (▶ Fig. 4.7, ▶ Fig. 4.8). However, all of them share common complications: an incomplete block necessitating conversion to GA or supplementation with peripheral nerve blocks. Neurapraxia can occur in up to 10% of all blocks and resolves within 6 weeks. Permanent nerve damage is rare and is seen in 1 in 3,000 to 5,000 cases. The sensation of high injection pressure indicates intraneural injections and warrants needle repositioning. There is also a risk of intravascular injection, which can result in systemic toxicity. Constant aspiration prevents this complication, which can result in seizures, arrhythmias, and death. Tourniquet pain will often be noted by the patient as the intercostobrachial nerve (T2) which innervates the posterolateral aspect of the arm is not part of the brachial plexus; this nerve should be blocked independently.

4.3.1 Axillary Blockade

This block is suitable for the forearm, wrist, and hand. The patient is supine with the arm abducted and externally rotated with the dorsum of the hand resting on the bed. The axillary artery is palpated in the axilla, the needle entry point is just lateral to the lateral border of the pectoralis major and superior to the axillary artery (▶ Fig. 4.7). Axillary blockade can be performed with nerve stimulation; however, block with ultrasound probe

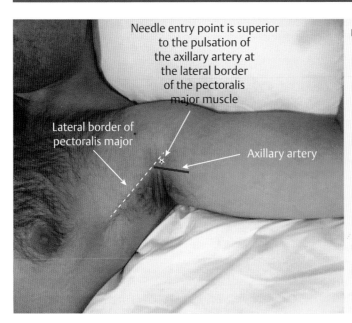

Needle entry point is superior to the pulsation of the axillary artery at the lateral border of the pectoralis major muscle

Lateral border of pectoralis major

Axillary artery

Fig. 4.7 Landmarks for axillary block.

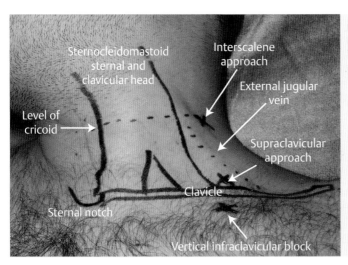

Sternocleidomastoid sternal and clavicular head

Interscalene approach

External jugular vein

Level of cricoid

Supraclavicular approach

Clavicle

Sternal notch

Vertical infraclavicular block

Fig. 4.8 Landmarks for supraclavicular block, interscalene block, and infraclavicular block.

allows visualization of the axillary artery, and the three main nerves to be blocked (radial, median, and ulnar).

4.3.2 Supraclavicular and Infraclavicular Blockade

The needle entry site is superior to the clavicle and just lateral to the point where the sternocleidomastoid is attached to the clavicle (▶ Fig. 4.8). This method can reliably block the entire arm, but

there is a higher risk of pneumothorax. The technique is best performed with ultrasound blockade helping the anesthetist to visualize the brachial plexus, subclavian artery, and the pleural cavity.

In the infraclavicular block, the sternal notch and the ventral apophysis of the acromion are marked. The midpoint between these two points is measured; the needle entry point is directly below the clavicle in a vertical direction. Ultrasound guidance can minimize the risk of pneumothorax.

4.3.3 Interscalene Blockade

This is the most cranial of the upper limb blocks. The needle is placed in the interscalene groove which lies between the anterior and the middle scalene. The cricoid cartilage at the level of C6 and lateral border of the sternomastoid muscle helps identify the interscalene groove. The technique can be performed with a nerve stimulator or ultrasound blockade. The interscalene block provides anesthesia for the shoulder, upper arm, and elbow.

Selected Readings

Chiu DT. Transthecal digital block: flexor tendon sheath used for anesthetic infusion. J Hand Surg Am. 1990; 15(3):471–477

First description of the utilization of the flexor tendon sheath as a site of local anesthetic injection in digital blocks. The author used the transthecal approach in 420 patients and injected 2 mL of lidocaine into the sheath at the level of the A1 pulley using a 25-gauge needle. Chiu advocated this technique as a viable alternative to the traditional digital nerve blockade, with similar speed and duration of anesthesia. He did not note any evidence of toxicity and only four patients in his cohort needed further supplementation of their anesthesia following the initial injection.

Low CK, Vartany A, Engstrom JW, Poncelet A, Diao E. Comparison of transthecal and subcutaneous single-injection digital block techniques. J Hand Surg Am. 1997; 22(5):901–905

Randomized double-blinded studies comparing the transthecal and single-injection subcutaneous technique on each index finger in a cohort of 20 healthy volunteers. Evaluation of efficacy of blockade was performed by measuring pain, light touch, and nerve conduction studies. The methods of anesthetic administration were similar with regard to the onset and duration of the anesthetic effect. Importantly, subcutaneous blocks were proven to be associated with less pain at the injection site both at the time of instillation and 24 hours later.

Low CK, Wong HP, Low YP. Comparison between single injection transthecal and subcutaneous digital blocks. J Hand Surg [Br]. 1997; 22(5):582–584

Randomized double-blinded study from orthopaedic department in Singapore comparing two different techniques of single-injection techniques in digital blocks: subcutaneous and intrathecal injections. A total of 3 mL of a mixture of lignocaine/bupivacaine was injected into 157 digits using the two techniques. Complete anesthesia was achieved in over 90% of cases in both groups with no significant differences in effectiveness, speed of onset, or duration of anesthetic effect.

Thorne C, Grabb WC. Grabb and Smith's Plastic Surgery. 7th ed. Philadelphia, PA: Wolters Kluwer/Lippincott Williams & Wilkins; 2014

Chapter 71 in this classic Plastic Surgery textbook depicts the various approaches to anesthesia of the upper limb. It provides a step-by-step description of the various brachial plexus and peripheral nerve blocks as well as the intravenous (Bier's block) technique. Chapter 12 in the same book provides an extensive description of the pharmacology of the individual agents used in locoregional anesthesia.

5 Nailbed Repair

Dariush Nikkhah, Jeremy Rodrigues

Keywords: nailbed repair, Seymour fracture

5.1 Nailbed Injuries

Pediatric nailbed injuries are commonplace in many hand surgery units (▶ Fig. 5.1). Adults can be operated on under local anesthesia, but in young children, general anesthesia is needed.

If there is evidence of subungual hematoma, or the nail has been partially avulsed, exploration and repair is usually warranted (▶ Fig. 5.2, ▶ Fig. 5.3, ▶ Fig. 5.4, ▶ Fig. 5.5). Many of these injuries have tuft fractures that can be managed conservatively.

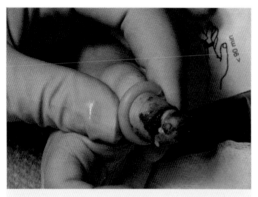

Fig. 5.1 Right thumb nailbed injury in a 2-year-old child.

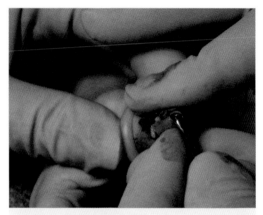

Fig. 5.2 Nail plate is lifted with Mitchell's trimmer; this prevents inadvertent removal of sterile matrix. After sufficient release, Stevens' tenotomy scissors can be used to lift off the nail plate.

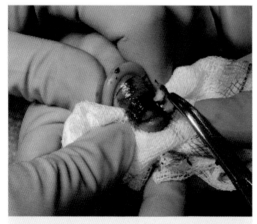

Fig. 5.3 The nail plate can then be grasped on one side with a mosquito clamp and peeled off slowly avoiding injury to the underlying sterile matrix.

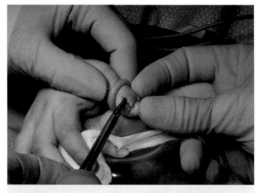

Fig. 5.4 Once the nailbed is washed, and hematoma is removed, one can repair the sterile matrix with 6.0 or 7.0 braided absorbable suture such as Vicryl Rapide. The sterile matrix is important for contact adherence. The new nail forms from the germinal matrix, which contributes 90% growth of the nail.

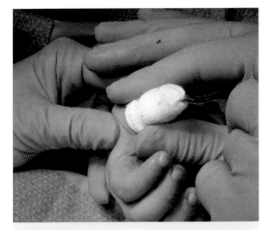

Fig. 5.5 Finger bob dressing applied after removal of tourniquet. Underneath this, a nonadherent silicone primary dressing is used as it will be left in situ for several days.

Some surgeons have advocated that the nail plate should not be placed back after repair, due to a possible higher risk of infection, although the nail plate can act as a splint for some fractures of the distal phalanx and may prevent the formation of synechiae. If replaced, the nail plate can be secured with a simple figure of 8 stitch using Vicryl Rapide. Tissue glue can cause problems with prolonged adherence of the old nail plate, in the author's experience.

5.2 Seymour Fracture

Displaced distal phalangeal fractures that involve the physis with an associated nailbed laceration

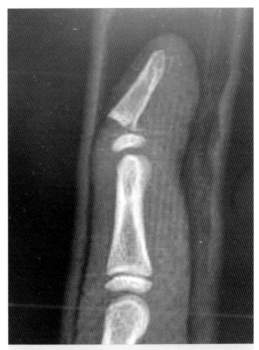

Fig. 5.6 Classical presentation of Seymour fracture with unopposed action of the flexor digitorum profundus (FDP) tendon.

are termed Seymour fractures (▶ Fig. 5.6). Clinically, these injuries present with a flexed posture of the distal phalanx almost resembling a mallet finger (▶ Fig. 5.7a,b). This is due to differences in insertions of the flexor and extensor tendon, with the former inserting into the metaphysis and the latter more proximally into the physis. Clinical

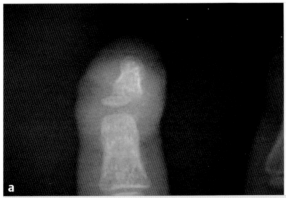
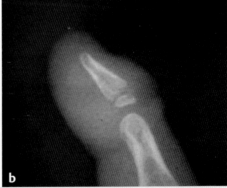

Fig. 5.7 (a,b) (Posteroanterior and lateral) More subtle presentation of Seymour fracture. There is an evidence of a displaced distal phalangeal physeal fracture.

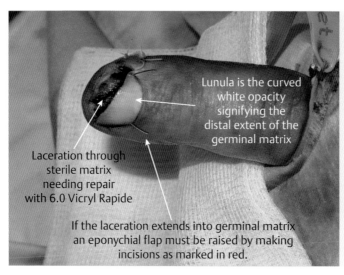

Fig. 5.8 Nailbed laceration through sterile matrix, nail plate does not need to be completely removed in this case. Red lines demonstrate incisions for eponychial flap that helps with repair of germinal matrix in more proximal injuries of the nailbed.

Lunula is the curved white opacity signifying the distal extent of the germinal matrix

Laceration through sterile matrix needing repair with 6.0 Vicryl Rapide

If the laceration extends into germinal matrix an eponychial flap must be raised by making incisions as marked in red.

Surgically, it is important to remove interposed soft tissue from the fracture site and then anatomical alignment of the fracture and physis can be achieved. It is often necessary to raise an eponychial flap to achieve adequate visualization of the fracture site (▶ Fig. 5.8). Once reduction is maintained, a single 0.9-mm Kirschner wire (K-wire) can be placed in a retrograde manner (▶ Fig. 5.9).

5.3 Rehabilitation after Nailbed Injuries

After operation, patients will spend the first 5 to 7 days in a bulky bandage. After this wound care, early motion of the digit (with K-wire protection, if required) and desensitization is important. The K-wire is removed at 3 to 4 weeks.

Selected Readings

Miranda BH, Vokshi I, Milroy CJ. Pediatric nailbed repair study: nail replacement increases morbidity. Plast Reconstr Surg. 2012; 129 (2):394e–396e

A retrospective single-center study of 111 cases of pediatric nailbed injuries. Study results suggest that replacement of the nail plate increases the risk of wound healing complications and risk of infection in patients younger than 16. This also translated to a significant increase in the number of outpatient visits and no improved outcomes in terms of cosmesis or function. As such, the authors advocate that nail plates be discarded intraoperatively and not used as splints for the underlying repair.

Roser SE, Gellman H. Comparison of nail bed repair versus nail trephination for subungual hematomas in children. J Hand Surg Am. 1999; 24(6):1166–1170

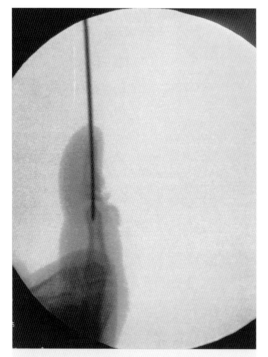

Fig. 5.9 Seymour fracture in ▶ Fig. 5.6 fixed with retrograde K-wire fixation.

presentation can be more subtle, however, with an avulsed nail plate and tenderness, which are the only clinical signs. A plain X-ray is important, as failure to identify a Seymour fracture may result in nail plate deformity, physeal arrest, or osteomyelitis.

Study comparing nail plate trephination versus formal nailbed repair in pediatric patients presenting with subungual hematomas. All cases of visible lacerations to the nailbed/perionychium were excluded and follow-up exceeded 2 years in all cases. Trephination was found to have the same long-term outcomes irrespective of the size of the hematoma, presence of bony injury, or age. It also resulted in savings of over one thousand dollars per case treated. The authors recommend that nailbed exploration is not warranted in children who present with subungual hematomas with no visible lacerations to the fingertip.

Seymour N. Juxta-epiphysial fracture of the terminal phalanx of the finger. J Bone Joint Surg Br. 1966; 48(2):347–349

Original description of the Seymour fracture with description of clinical/radiological characteristics and treatment principles. A description of the classic appearance of the transverse juxta-epiphyseal fracture with unopposed pull of the flexor digitorum profundus (FDP) tendon on the distal bony segment. The author recommends that the fracture is managed with manipulation of the fracture segments by applying a hyperextension force to the distal phalanx and subsequent splinting of the fracture with nail plate replacement and a Zimmer splint holding the distal interphalangeal joint (DIPJ) in extension.

Sierakowski A, Gardiner MD, Jain A, Greig AV, Nail bed INJury Analysis (NINJA) Collaborative Group. Surgical treatment of paediatric nail bed injuries in the United Kingdom: Surgeon and patient priorities for future research. J Plast Reconstr Aesthet Surg. 2016; 69(2):286–288

Study consisting of three individual components. Firstly, a questionnaire enquiring about nailbed repair practice was collected from a total of 116 surgeons in the United Kingdom. Secondly, a retrospective analysis of a month's worth of nailbed injuries was performed (54 nailbed injuries in total). Lastly, a survey was sent out to parents of children with nailbed injuries, enquiring about their perception of the injury and outcomes. Important findings of the study included: 96% of the health care professionals replaced the nail plate following repair of the nailbed; 52% of all injuries had an associated fracture of the distal phalanx. Parents were mostly concerned regarding the regrowth of the nail and risk of infection.

6 Hand Infections

Dariush Nikkhah

Keywords: flexor sheath infection, flexor sheath washout, fight bite, paronychia

tions with subcutaneous purulence may need to be managed with an open approach using broad mid-lateral flaps to prevent flap necrosis.

6.1 Flexor Sheath Infection

Flexor sheath infections are heralded by Kanavel's signs: fusiform swelling, flexed posture to digit, pain over flexor sheath, and pain on passive extension (▶ Fig. 6.1). These infections should be treated with emergent washout to avoid chronic hand dysfunction and in severe cases amputation.

Early presentations without subcutaneous purulence can be washed with a closed technique and can be given intravenous antibiotics. Later presenta-

6.2 Flexor Sheath Washout

Once the flexor sheath is opened proximally, a green cannula with the metallic introducer is placed underneath the A1 pulley. The introducer maintains rigidity and prevents kinking of the plastic sheath. Sometimes due to swelling it is necessary to vent the A1 pulley to gain access. Distal access is made through the A5 pulley. If the surgeon remains midline, neurovascular structures will remain safe (▶ Fig. 6.2, ▶ Fig. 6.3, ▶ Fig. 6.4, ▶ Fig. 6.5).

It is also important to lift the flexor digitorum superficialis (FDS) and flexor digitorum profundus (FDP) with a tendon hook to break up loculations and adhesions particularly if the patient is returning to theater for a second debridement (▶ Fig. 6.6).

In cases where there is subcutaneous purulence or a closed technique has failed to improve the infection, an open approach is advised (▶ Fig. 6.7, ▶ Fig. 6.8). Flaps should be kept broad to prevent tip necrosis and tendon exposure. A midlateral incision has a key advantage over a Bruner-type incision as the flap can cover the flexor tendons when the wounds are left open. Bruner flaps need to be at least tacked together to prevent retraction and tendon exposure.

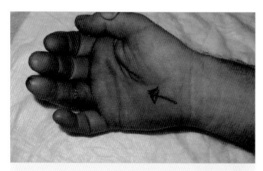

Fig. 6.1 Classical presentation of a flexor sheath infection in the ring finger. Grossly swollen digit with foreign body puncture wound.

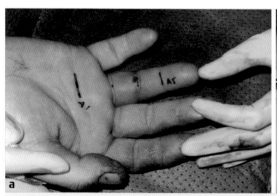
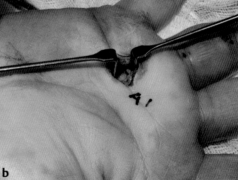

Fig. 6.2 (a,b) Markings over A1 and A5 pulley for closed irrigation technique and blunt dissection down to A1 pulley and flexor sheath.

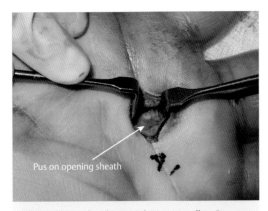

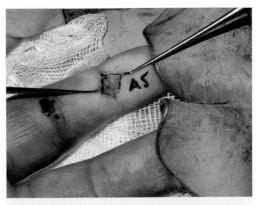

Fig. 6.3 Flexor sheath opened over A1 pulley. Pus identified and swabbed for microbiology to determine antibiotic sensitivities.

Fig. 6.4 Blunt dissection down to A5 pulley for distal access of flexor sheath, care here not to injure the digital nerves as they can be very superficial.

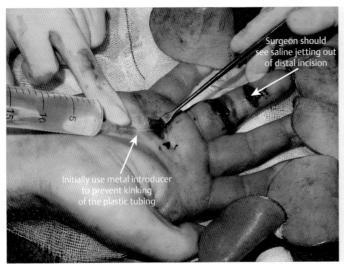

Fig. 6.5 A green cannula with a metallic introducer is used to irrigate from the A1 to A5 pulley. The "fountain sign" can be seen with saline coming out from the A5 pulley.

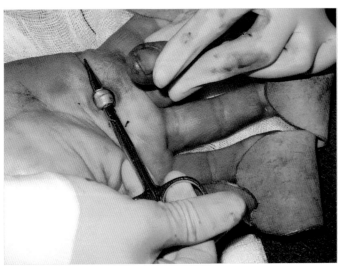

Fig. 6.6 Often in flexor sheath infections the FDS and FDP tendons become adherent and the surgeon must lift them up to break up loculations and adhesions. This helps facilitate closed catheter irrigation. The green cannula can also be placed between the FDS and FDP tendons for closed catheter irrigation.

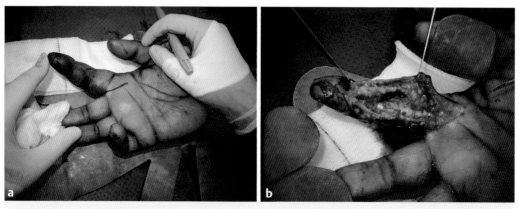

Fig. 6.7 (a,b) Midlateral open approach is warranted in cases where there is subcutaneous purulence over the entire digit.

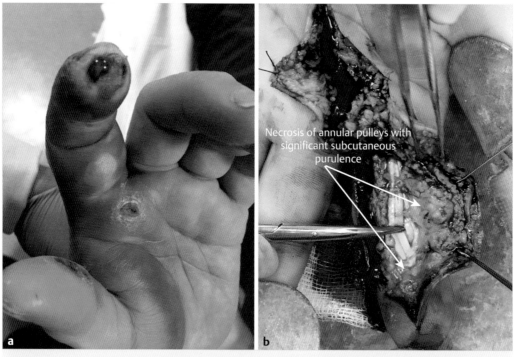

Fig. 6.8 (a,b) Similar case demonstrating severe flexor sheath infection with subcutaneous purulence. There is obliteration of the annular pulleys. A closed technique would not address the infection.

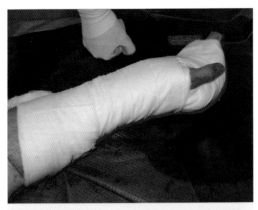

Fig. 6.9 Soft band is wrapped around Betadine-soaked gauze and Jelonet before plaster of Paris application.

Wounds should be left open and dressed with Betadine-soaked gauze over Jelonet and a plaster of Paris in the position of safe immobilization (▶ Fig. 6.9, ▶ Fig. 6.10). The injured hand should be placed in a high-arm sling to reduce edema.

6.3 Fight Bite

These injuries are common presentations in the emergency department and occur when a clenched fist hits an opponent's tooth. The bacterial flora of the opponent's tooth can enter the joint and result in septic arthritis.

Patients usually present, as in the case demonstrated, with erythema, severe pain on joint movement, and pus extruding from the wound (▶ Fig. 6.11). These patients need emergent exploration and washout of the joint to prevent joint destruction (▶ Fig. 6.12, ▶ Fig. 6.13).

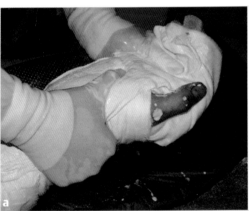
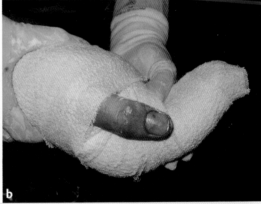

Fig. 6.10 (a,b) The surgeon must place the hand in the functional position with the wrist in 30 degrees and the MCPJ at 60 to 70 degrees. This arrangement places the collaterals in maximal stretch.

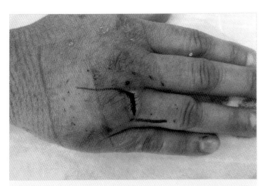

Fig. 6.11 Laceration over extensor zone 5 after a fight bite. Area of erythema marked with dotted line.

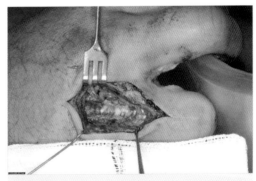

Fig. 6.12 The wound is extended longitudinally in these injuries and the MCPJ is always visualized by partially dividing the sagittal band.

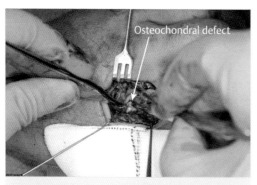

Fig.6.13 The surgeon is then able to see an osteochondral defect on axial traction of the digit, which needs saline irrigation and curettage of the bone. (Reproduced with permission from Nikkhah D, Vijayan R, Bhat W. The significance of bone abrasions in fight bite injuries: beware of the osteochondral defect. Hand Surg. 2015 Oct;20(3):488.)

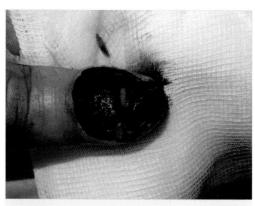

Fig.6.15 Decompression of pus after removal of the nail plate.

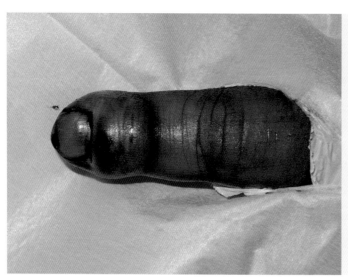

Fig.6.14 Paronychia infection.

6.4 Paronychia

These cases present with pus in the paronychial space (▶ Fig. 6.14). Some remove the nail plate partially; however, it is best to remove it in its entirety to prevent reaccumulation or incomplete release of pus in the paronychial space (▶ Fig. 6.15).

A curvilinear incision is firstly made over the paronychia over the site of maximal fluctuance. The entire procedure can be performed under ring block. Often there is epidermolysis and the infection can cause subcutaneous purulence across the length of the digit. Only cases of late presentation can result in osteomyelitis and even terminalization of the digit.

6.5 Rehabilitation after Hand Infections

After initial debridement and washout, these injuries need to be placed in a volar resting splint in the position of safe immobilization. Once infection has been controlled, the patient should be removed from the splint and early active and passive range-of-motion exercises should be started. Without early hand therapy, this patient group is at high risk of stiffness and tendon adhesions.

Selected Readings

Giladi AM, Malay S, Chung KC. A systematic review of the management of acute pyogenic flexor tenosynovitis. J Hand Surg Eur Vol. 2015; 40(7):720–728

A systematic review of a total of 763 cases of pyogenic flexor tenosynovitis (PFT) in a total of 28 studies. Variations in surgical approach and medical therapy were considered. Mean follow-up of patients was 20 months. Amputation rates were found to be higher in cases of PFT in patients with systemic illness such as diabetes, peripheral vascular disease, and renal insufficiency. Range of motion was greater when broad-spectrum antibiotics were used alongside surgical washout. Functional outcomes were also superior in catheter irrigation of the flexor sheath compared with open washout, which may result from the reduced iatrogenic injury to the flexor sheath in the closed technique.

Nikkhah D, Vijayan R, Bhat W. The significance of bone abrasions in fight bite injuries: beware of the osteochondral defect. Hand Surg. 2015; 20(3):488

Letter highlighting the importance of proper visualization of metacarpophalangeal joint (MCPJ) surfaces in cases of fight bite injury. Even when radiographs are normal, it is important to explore the joint and mechanically debride areas of sequestrum or osteochondral defects as these will later serve as a nidus for infection, which could result in osteomyelitis and even amputation. The joint can be opened up by getting the assistant to apply axial traction to the digit—this will allow for the introduction of instruments necessary for debridement of bone into the confined space.

Shewring DJ, Trickett RW, Subramanian KN, Hnyda R. The management of clenched fist 'fight bite' injuries of the hand. J Hand Surg Eur Vol. 2015; 40(8):819–824

Prospective study covering a 4-year period in a single center; 159 fight bite injuries involving the joints of the hand were included into the study; 80% of bites involved the MCPJ, with the remaining 20% involving the proximal interphalangeal joint (PIPJ). MCPJ injury was found to be associated with better outcomes than PIPJ injury. The latter had significant functional impairments in over 40% of cases, some of which necessitated arthrodesis or amputation. The authors advocate a tendon splitting approach when accessing the MCPJ as this avoids damage to the sagittal band mechanism.

Zubowicz VN, Gravier M. Management of early human bites of the hand: a prospective randomized study. Plast Reconstr Surg. 1991; 88(1):111–114

Prospective randomized study to determine optimal treatment in early human bites. A total of 48 patients who presented within 24 hours of injury and had no evidence of active infection or joint involvement were included. Debridement and wound irrigation alone resulted in an almost 50% chance of developing an infection. No infections were noted in the group receiving the same wound care as well as an oral antibiotic. The cost–benefit analysis demonstrated that in a sensible patient with an uncomplicated human bite, debridement and irrigation in the emergency department followed by oral antibiotics is the most effective solution.

7 Flexor Tendon Repair

Dariush Nikkhah, Wojciech Konczalik

Keywords: flexor tendon repair, early active mobilization, flexor tendon rehabilitation

7.1 Flexor Tendon Repair

The case illustrates a patient who grasped a knife with a clenched fist and subsequently has multiple zone 2 flexor tendon divisions (► Fig. 7.1). These injuries can be time consuming to repair and require technical skill and appropriate hand therapy. Single-digit flexor tendon injuries can be repaired under local anesthetic and adrenaline technique; however, in multitendon injury, as in the case above, general anesthetic is supplemented with regional anesthetic and tourniquet.

Anatomically, these injuries are divided into five zones. Zone 1 injuries occur distal to the flexor digitorum superficialis (FDS) insertion (► Fig. 7.2, ► Fig. 7.3). If the flexor digitorum profundus (FDP)

tendon becomes detached from the bone, a number of techniques have been described to reattach the tendon to bone. These range from Mitek mini anchor, pullout technique with button, and transosseous

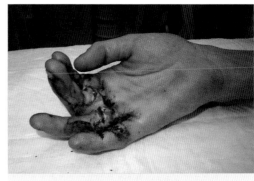

Fig. 7.1 Multiple flexor zone 2 tendon injuries after grasping a knife with a clenched hand.

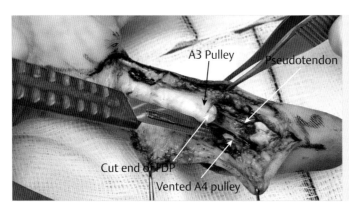

Fig. 7.2 100% division of FDP tendon at zone 1. Note the venting of A4 pulley with preservation of the A3 pulley. There is also evidence of pseudotendon formation.

A3 Pulley

Pseudotendon

Cut end of FDP

Vented A4 pulley

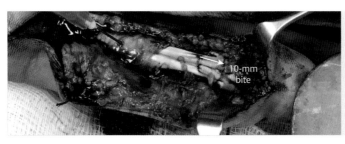

Fig. 7.3 After repair with a four-strand 3.0 round-bodied Prolene modified Kessler core stitch and 6.0 Prolene continuous epitendinous repair.

10-mm bite

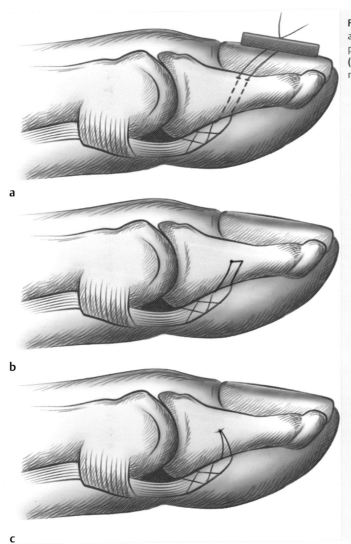

Fig. 7.4 Illustration of Mitek mini anchor repair, transosseous repairs, pullout repair with button. **(a)** Button pullout. **(b)** Transosseous repair. **(c)** Mitek mini anchor repair.

a

b

c

repairs (▸ Fig. 7.4 a–c). Zone 2 has its distal boundary at the FDS insertion and proximal boundary at the distal palmar crease. Zone 2 was known as *no man's land* and had poor outcomes historically, until Kleinert popularized direct repair with postoperative rehabilitation exercises. Zone 3 injuries occur in the palm, zone 4 in the carpal tunnel, and zone 5 in the wrist and forearm.

In the case illustrated earlier, a midlateral incision was performed to repair the damaged structures in zone 2 (▸ Fig. 7.5, ▸ Fig. 7.6, ▸ Fig. 7.7,

▸ Fig. 7.8, ▸ Fig. 7.9, ▸ Fig. 7.10, ▸ Fig. 7.11, ▸ Fig. 7.12). Generally, a four-strand modified Kessler repair is performed for the core stitch to minimize the gapping and an epitendinous repair provides an additional 25% strength to the tendon repair (▸ Fig. 7.13, ▸ Fig. 7.14). At least a 10-mm bite should be taken with the core suture to provide optimal strength. The blood supply to the flexor tendons is dorsal with a relatively avascular volar zone. One should try to preserve the pulleys, mainly the A2 and A4, but not at the cost of

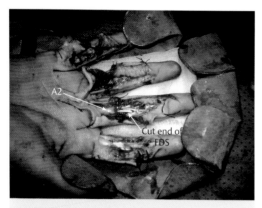

Fig. 7.5 To save operative time, all digits are opened through midlateral incisions and flaps are tacked back with silk.

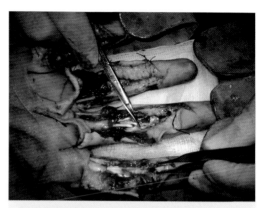

Fig. 7.6 The tenotomy scissors demonstrate Camper's chiasm. The middle finger has 100% division of the FDS at Camper's chiasm and the FDP has retracted back proximal to the A2 pulley.

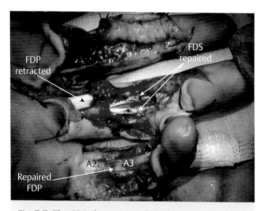

Fig. 7.7 The FDS slips are small, and in this case, these are repaired with a 3.0 round-bodied Prolene suture using a horizontal mattress core stitch. In some cases, it is not possible to repair both FDS slips or the FDP tendon will not be able to glide sufficiently.

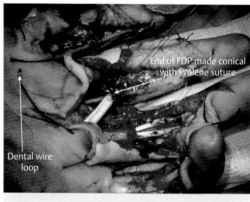

Fig. 7.8 A small window is made in the sheath proximal to the A2 pulley and the FDP tendon is retrieved. To pass it under the A2 pulley, a dental wire is used to retrieve the tendon.

limiting tendon glide. Some surgeons advocate venting to facilitate glide after repair. Indeed, sometimes it is necessary to vent the entire A4 pulley for tendon repair; as long as the A2 pulley is preserved, tendon bowstringing is minimized. Furthermore, in some cases it is not possible to repair both FDS tendons as this will impede FDP excursion, and increase the work of flexion. A dorsal plaster of Paris is used to protect the repair at the end of the procedure (▶ Fig. 7.15).

The same principles of tendon repair apply with the flexor pollicis longus (FPL) repair; however, access is best achieved through Bruner-type incisions (▶ Fig. 7.16, ▶ Fig. 7.17). The FPL can retract to the carpal tunnel and the dental wire technique for retrieval is useful (▶ Fig. 7.18). Once retrieved, the FPL should be repaired with a four-strand modified Kessler and epitendinous repair with preservation of the oblique pulley to prevent bowstringing (▶ Fig. 7.19).

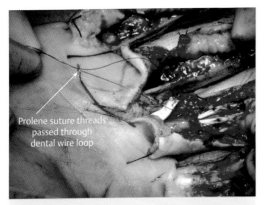

Fig. 7.9 Retrieval of retracted FDP with dental wire. A suture is passed twice through the tip of the FDP to make it conical so it can be easily passed through the pulleys. The suture is then passed through the dental wire loop.

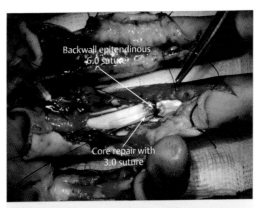

Fig. 7.11 Repair starts with a back wall 6.0 round-bodied Prolene and then a four-strand 3.0 Prolene round-bodied Kessler repair.

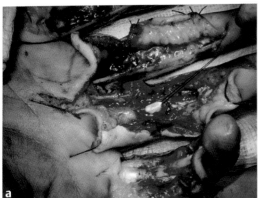
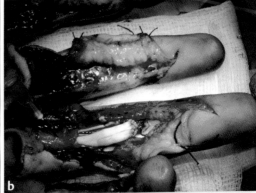

Fig. 7.10 (a,b) The FDP is retrieved and then anchored with a blue needle.

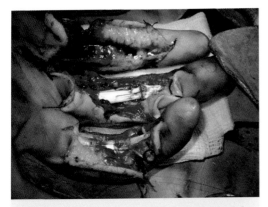

Fig. 7.12 The final repair is tested 10 times to check for gapping at the repair site. In this case, the A3 and A4 pulleys were vented.

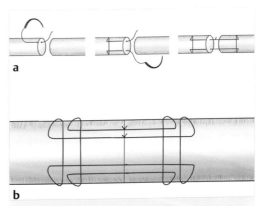

Fig. 7.13 Illustration of (a) the modified Kessler core stitch and (b) a four-strand modified Kessler repair.

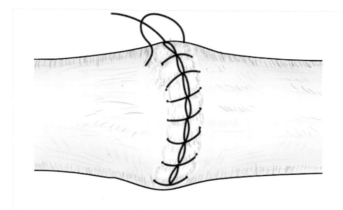

Fig. 7.14 Illustration of epitendinous repair.

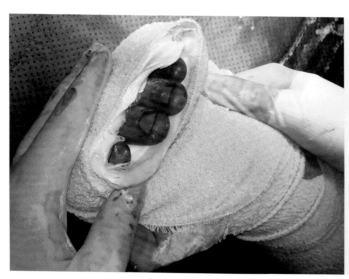

Fig. 7.15 A plaster of Paris dorsal blocking splint is used to protect the repair in the first 3 days before it is changed to a thermoplastic splint (wrist 0 degree flexion, metacarpophalangeal joint [MCPJ] 40 degrees' flexion, IPJ straight).

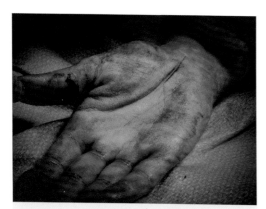

Fig. 7.16 Access is marked with Bruner-type incision, in some cases the carpal tunnel needs to be accessed to retrieve the FPL tendon.

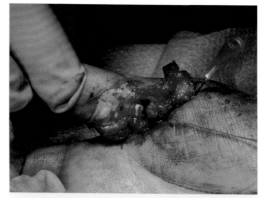

Fig. 7.17 If the tendon has retracted back slightly, a skin hook can be used to retrieve it. The same principles apply with a back wall 6.0 Prolene and it is always necessary in FPL repairs to use a four-strand core repair.

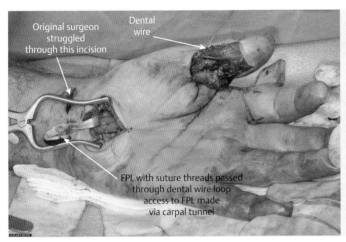

Original surgeon struggled through this incision

Dental wire

FPL with suture threads passed through dental wire loop access to FPL made via carpal tunnel

Fig. 7.18 Retrieval of FPL with dental wire. The original surgeon had struggled to retrieve FPL through a separate incision in wrist.

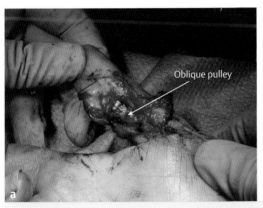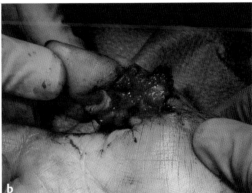

Oblique pulley

a b

Fig. 7.19 (a,b) The oblique pulley is preserved and the FPL tendon is tested with passive flexion for any catching or obstruction of glide.

7.2 Rehabilitation after Flexor Tendon Repair (Adult and Pediatric)

Hand therapy should start 3 to 5 days postoperatively. A dorsal blocking splint will need to be worn at all the times for 4 weeks and then part time for 2 to 4 weeks (▶ Fig. 7.20). Patients are given extensive advice and education as removing the splint too early will result in a high risk of snapping the tendon.

It will take 12 weeks until the tendon will fully heal and until the patient can resume heavy activities by the hand.

The approach adopted by most of the UK centers is early active mobilization in a dorsal blocking splint (▶ Fig. 7.21). Four-strand repairs allow the therapists to glide the tendons earlier and reduce the risk of adhesions without increasing the rupture rate. Passive flexion of the fingers and then early active glide of the repaired tendons are essential. Extension of the digit to the splint also limits flexion deformities of the interphalangeal joints (IPJs).

Children under 5 years should be treated in a bulky boxing glove bandage for 4 to 6 weeks. Children of school age generally cope with an early active motion regime but have a bar or cover on the volar aspect to prevent function.

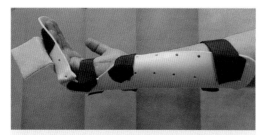

Fig. 7.20 Dorsal blocking thermoplastic splint.

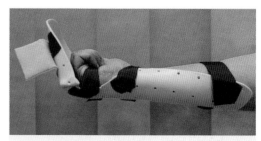

Fig. 7.21 Early active mobilization.

Selected Readings

Cooper L, Khor W, Burr N, Sivakumar B. Flexor tendon repairs in children: outcomes from a specialist tertiary centre. J Plast Reconstr Aesthet Surg. 2015; 68(5):717–723

The authors describe their functional outcomes after early active mobilization in a pediatric population. Their rehabilitation protocol included boxing glove immobilization (<5 years), dorsal blocking splint and cage (5–10 years), or dorsal blocking splint ± cage (10–16 years). On 63 fingers and 99 tendons good/excellent results were obtained in 82% of patients using the total active mobilization method of the American Society for Surgery of the Hand. Only one tendon rupture was reported.

Cullen KW, Tolhurst P, Lang D, Page RE. Flexor tendon repair in zone 2 followed by controlled active mobilisation. J Hand Surg [Br]. 1989; 14(4):392–395

British study describing an early mobilization protocol for flexor tendon injuries. A total of 70 tendons in 38 patients were included into the study and they were followed up over a 2-year period. Good range of motion with low complication rates were achieved. Exercises (both active and passive movements) are initiated after a period of 48 hours, when the initial postoperative inflammation subsides. The splint is discontinued at 4 to 6 weeks and progressive resistive exercise and heavier hand use are instituted at 8 weeks with full return to activity at 12 weeks of postsurgery.

Huq S, George S, Boyce DE. Zone 1 flexor tendon injuries: a review of the current treatment options for acute injuries. J Plast Reconstr Aesthet Surg. 2013; 66(8):1023–1031

This review discusses the different treatment options for zone 1 flexor tendon injuries where the tendon has avulsed from the distal phalanx. The traditional button pullout technique has been associated with significant morbidity and therefore alternative methods have been developed. Internal suture techniques and bone anchor techniques are described and outcome data show low complication rates.

King IC, Nikkhah D. Re: Wong J. and McGrouther D. A. Minimizing trauma over 'no man's land' for flexor tendon retrieval. J Hand Surg Eur Vol. 2015; 40(4):428–430

Technical paper describing a method for retrieval of retracted flexor tendons with minimal disruption of the pulley system. The proximal end is identified in the wound and a 3/0 Ethibond suture on a round-bodied needle is passed through the stump twice. A folded dental wire is then inserted at the site of the distal stump and passed in a retrograde fashion through the flexor sheath and underneath the pulleys to reach the proximal tendon. The long ends of the Ethibond suture are then looped around the dental wire, which is then gently retracted, allowing for the delivery of the tendon beneath the pulley system in preparation for repair. This solution is technically easier than the previously described technique utilizing pediatric catheters, and it is also less expensive.

Kleinert HE, Kutz JE, Ashbell TS, Martinez E. Primary repair of lacerated flexor tendons in "no man's land". J Bone Joint Surg Am. 1967; 49A:577

This seminal paper represented the first large series of primary repair of flexor tendons in flexor zone 2 followed by an early passive motion protocol. About 87% of patients treated had good to excellent results based on flexion and extension.

Kwai Ben I, Elliot D. "Venting" or partial lateral release of the A2 and A4 pulleys after repair of zone 2 flexor tendon injuries. J Hand Surg [Br]. 1998; 23(5):649–654

This article discusses the authors' experience of lateral release or venting of the A2 and A4 pulleys. In a series of 126 repairs, 64% of repairs required venting of one or the other pulley. It was necessary to vent the A4 pulley between 10 and 100% of its length in 56% of repairs and to vent the distal edge of the A2 pulley in 8% of fingers.

Savage R. In vitro studies of a new method of flexor tendon repair. J Hand Surg [Br]. 1985; 10(2):135–141

A description of flexor tendon repair allowing for better grasping of the tendon relative to commonly used techniques. This core suture allows for a strong six-stranded repair, which increases the tensile strength threefold relative to other two-strand repairs and minimizes gapping by over 90%. The blood supply of the tendon is not significantly constricted in this technique and due to its large bite size, it allows for early mobilization even during the inflammatory phase of healing when the tendon stumps become edematous and friable.

Savage R. The search for the ideal tendon repair in zone 2: strand number, anchor points and suture thickness. J Hand Surg Eur Vol. 2014; 39(1):20–29

Review of mechanical factors involved in surgical tendon repair. Placement of anchor points, number of core strands, size of suture material, and the use of epitendinous repair techniques were reviewed. A two-strand repair using the modified Kessler technique combined with simple epitendinous repair had a rupture rate of approximately 10% and therefore was not recommended by the author as a satisfactory method to repair a flexor tendon. The author concludes that optimal repair is achieved by means of a four- or six-strand core repair and should be further supplemented by a peripheral suture, which prevents gapping and smoothens out the bulky aspects of the repair.

Tang JB. Release of the A4 pulley to facilitate zone II flexor tendon repair. J Hand Surg Am. 2014; 39(11):2300–2307

The A4 pulley is the narrowest part of the flexor sheath. Disrupted tendon ends are usually swollen and therefore it can make passage of the FDP tendon difficult. If the A2 and A3 pulleys are intact, the entire A4 pulley can be vented through a lateral incision to accommodate repair.

8 Extensor Tendon Repair

Dariush Nikkhah, Amir H. Sadr

Keywords: extensor tendon repair, rehabilitation after extensor repair, Silfverskiöld repair

8.1 Extensor Tendon Repair

The patient presented with a glass laceration over the thumb metacarpophalangeal joint (MCPJ) and had an inability to extend the thumb on the retropulsion test (▶ Fig. 8.1). They were booked for local anesthetic exploration and repair of the extensor pollicis longus (EPL) (▶ Fig. 8.2, ▶ Fig. 8.3, ▶ Fig. 8.4, ▶ Fig. 8.5, ▶ Fig. 8.6). Most distal extensors can be done under local anesthetic; however, once you get to proximal zones 6 and 7, it can become trickier under local anesthetic as the tendons retract.

Extensor tendon injuries are more common than flexor tendon injuries due to their less protected anatomical location. Some surgeons underestimate the management of these injuries which require the same skill and attention to

detail as flexor tendon surgery to avoid poor results. Verdan classified extensor tendon injuries in zones 1 to 9. The odd numbers 1, 3, 5, and 7 lie over the joints with zone 1 lying over the distal interphalangeal joint (DIPJ). The importance of this is that in zones 1 to 3 the tendon is flatter and may not easily accommodate a core stitch. Ideally, if it is possible, one should do a core repair with an additional epitendinous repair. The Silfverskiöld repair is a useful technique in flat extensor tendons and provides a strong repair (▶ Fig. 8.7, ▶ Fig. 8.8, ▶ Fig. 8.9, ▶ Fig. 8.10, ▶ Fig. 8.11).

Note: In zones 1 and 2, most of the proximal pull on the terminal extensor comes from the lumbricals via the lateral bands. Thus, flexing the digit at the MCPJ and proximal interphalangeal joint (PIPJ) can facilitate a tight repair by detensioning the lateral bands. Conversely, in zone 3 (and more proximally), extending the digit relaxes the proximal extensor digitorum communis (EDC) tendon to aid suture repair of the central slip.

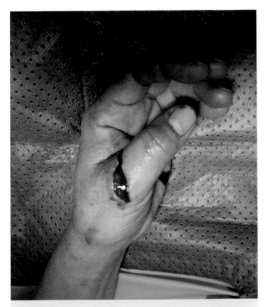

Fig. 8.1 Thumb demonstrates an abnormal posture suggestive of EPL division.

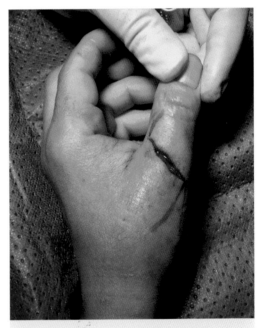

Fig. 8.2 Access is gained with broad longitudinal flaps.

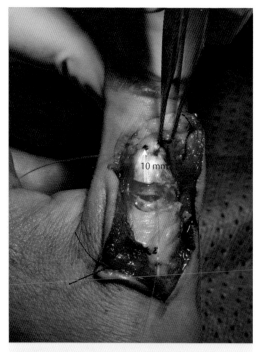

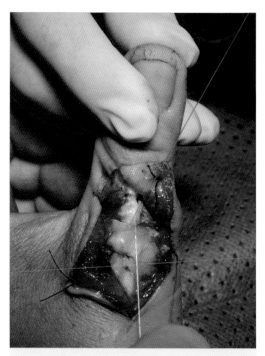

Fig. 8.3 The extensor tendon is marked with ink approximately 10 mm. This reminds the surgeon to take appropriate bites for the core suture.

Fig. 8.4 A two-strand core 3.0 PDS modified Kessler is used initially and tied. We advocate PDS use over Prolene to prevent the nonabsorbable knots of the Prolene irritating the thinner dorsal skin.

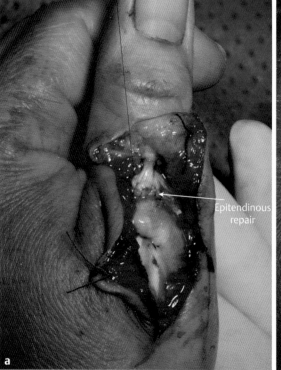

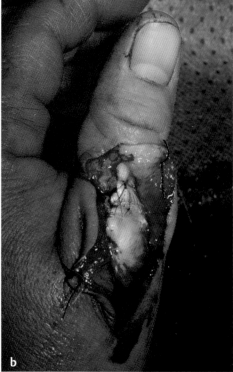

Fig. 8.5 (a,b) This is followed by a continuous 6.0 epitendinous PDS. An alternative complex epitendinous suture is a Silfverskiöld repair that provides additional strength compared to simple epitendinous repairs.

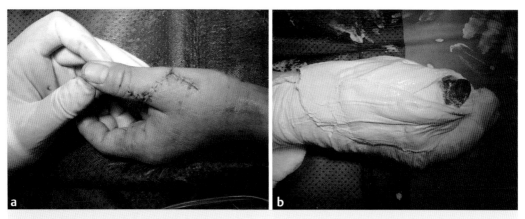

Fig. 8.6 (a,b) Final closure with 5.0 Vicryl Rapide and EPL repair is protected in forearm-based thumb spica-based plaster of Paris.

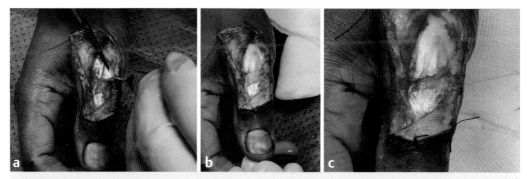

Fig. 8.7 (a–c) EPL division, tendon ends are first cleaned before repair. Back wall epitendinous repair is done with 5.0 Prolene. This draws the tendon together and is a very useful technique especially when there is a large gap. It enables easier core stitch placement.

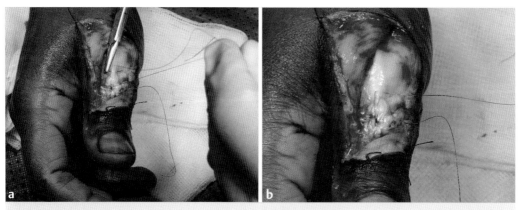

Fig. 8.8 (a,b) Core suture of modified Kessler 3.0 PDS is then followed by Silfverskiöld cross-stitch repair where the surgeon stitches toward himself or herself.

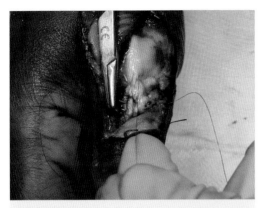

Fig. 8.9 The surgeon sutures toward himself or herself in order to complete the repair.

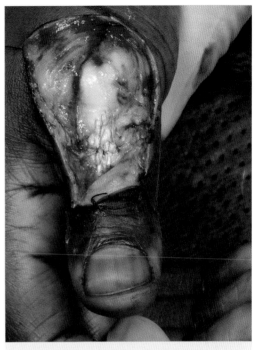

Fig. 8.10 Completed Silfverskiöld cross-stitch repair.

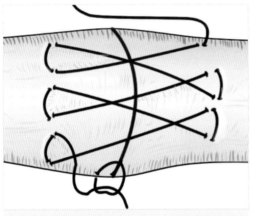

Fig. 8.11 Illustration of Silfverskiöld cross-stitch repair.

Zone 9, which includes muscle belly, is best repaired with either Vicryl horizontal mattress sutures or a Monocryl pulley stitch.

8.2 Rehabilitation after Extensor Tendon Repair: Zones 5 to 8 and Thumbs

Patients should be referred to the hand therapist 3 to 5 days postoperation in a volar plaster of Paris splint (► Fig. 8.12). Rehabilitation for well-repaired

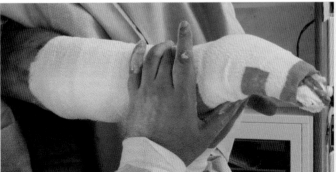

Fig. 8.12 Volar plaster of Paris splint after EDC tendon repair. Wrist: 40 degrees' extension, MP joint: 20 degrees' flexion, IPJ: straight.

extensors has progressed in the last 10 years and early motion techniques are now utilized in most UK centers rather than a static regime.

These tendons are protected in a splint for 4 to 8 weeks, but the splintage used will vary on the extent of the injury. Most centers utilize the Norwich regime or Merritt regime for their rehabilitation. Normal activities without a splint can be resumed around 6 to 8 weeks depending on tendon glide and motion. Heavier activities can resume at 8 to 12 weeks (▶ Fig. 8.13).

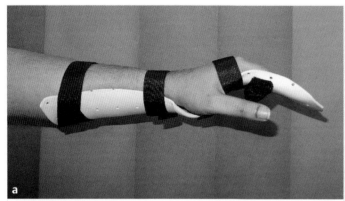

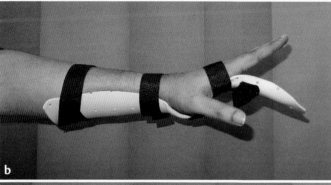

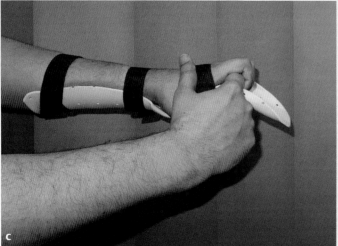

Fig. 8.13 (a–c) Extensor tendon early motion regime with repair protected in volar thermoplastic splint.

8.3 Rehabilitation Post Central Slip Repair: Zones 3 to 4

These are treated very differently from more proximal extensor tendon repairs. Most UK centers now treat surgically repaired central slip injuries with a short arc motion regime where an early glide of the PIPJ of up to 40 degrees is acceptable to prevent tethering in zone 4.

Selected Readings

Carl HD, Forst R, Schaller P. Results of primary extensor tendon repair in relation to the zone of injury and pre-operative outcome estimation. Arch Orthop Trauma Surg. 2007; 127(2): 115–119

Prospective study evaluating the functional outcomes following extensor tendon repair depending on the anatomical location of the injury. A total of 203 extensor tendon repairs were grouped according to Verdan's anatomical zones. A standard method of tendon repair and rehabilitation was used in all cases. The study found that functional outcome was lower in injuries to zones 3 and 6 and this was thought to be directly related to the higher incidence of complex injuries in these areas with concomitant soft-tissue and bony injury. The authors conclude that these cases may be better managed with static immobilisation to allow for more time for the soft-tissue envelope overlying the tendon repair site to fully heal.

Chow JA, Dovelle S, Thomes LJ, Ho PK, Saldana J. A comparison of results of extensor tendon repair followed by early controlled mobilisation versus static immobilisation. J Hand Surg [Br]. 1989; 14(1):18–20

Comparative study of early controlled mobilization and static immobilization rehabilitation protocols. All patients managed in the former manner demonstrated excellent functional recovery at 6 weeks. Static splints did not achieve satisfactory results in 30% of cases and had a higher propensity for extensor lag and adhesions requiring tenolysis. Early controlled motion achieved better outcomes with regard to improved grip strength and pulp-to-palm distance. The authors recommend the use of static splints only in cases where issues with compliance exist, as this regimen has improved therapy adherence.

O'Broin ES, Earley MJ, Smyth H, Hooper AC. Absorbable sutures in tendon repair. A comparison of PDS with Prolene in rabbit tendon repair. J Hand Surg [Br]. 1995; 20(4):505–508

This animal study demonstrated that there was no significant difference between polydioxanone (PDS) and Prolene in the first critical weeks of tendon healing. As PDS is absorbable, it avoids the risks of foreign implantation.

Sylaidis P, Youatt M, Logan A. Early active mobilization for extensor tendon injuries. The Norwich regime. J Hand Surg [Br]. 1997; 22 (5):594–596

Description of the commonly employed Norwich rehabilitation regime in extensor tendon injury. The regime relies on the principles of controlled active mobilization without dynamic splinting. The authors describe 37 extensor tendon injuries rehabilitated in this fashion with over 85% of these cases obtaining good or excellent function within 6 weeks of repair. The regimen obviates the need for dynamic splinting which can be cumbersome and difficult to manage. A static splint allowing controlled mobilization is applied within 48 hours of surgery and the patient commences range-of-motion exercises, which are to be performed every hour. The hand remains in a custom splint for 1 month, and after this time the splint is weaned until it is only worn during the night. The patient is allowed to perform light activities and over the course of the next 2 months gradually returns to normal levels of activity.

9 Closed Tendon Ruptures

Dariush Nikkhah, Robert Pearl

Keywords: tendon transfer, closed flexor digitorum profundus (FDP) rupture, Leddy Packer, Mitek, extensor indicis proprius (EIP) transfer

9.1 Extensor Indicis Proprius to Extensor Pollicis Longus Tendon Transfer

Closed rupture of extensor pollicis longus (EPL) at the wrist is the most common attrition tendon rupture. There is normally a history of distal radius fracture, often relatively undisplaced, and sometimes decades earlier. Direct repair is not possible and an extensor indicis proprius (EIP) to EPL transfer is an effective treatment.

The patient shown in ▶ Fig. 9.1 presented to the hand trauma clinic with an inability to extend the thumb. She had been managed conservatively in cast for 8 weeks for a distal radius fracture (▶ Fig. 9.2). Clinical examination confirmed a ruptured EPL tendon. An EIP to EPL transfer was performed under regional anesthetic (▶ Fig. 9.3, ▶ Fig. 9.4, ▶ Fig. 9.5, ▶ Fig. 9.6, ▶ Fig. 9.7). The EPL which lies in the third extensor compartment is thought to undergo ischemia due to edema which consequently results in tendon necrosis and rupture.

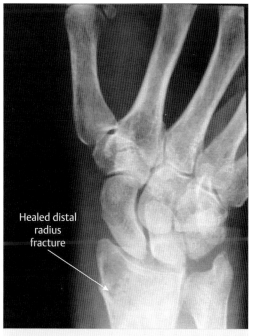

Healed distal radius fracture

Fig. 9.2 This radiograph demonstrates a healed distal radius fracture in the same patient.

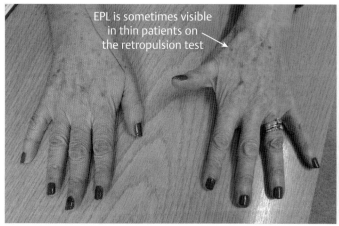

EPL is sometimes visible in thin patients on the retropulsion test

Fig. 9.1 The patient has an inability to extend the right thumb on the retropulsion test.

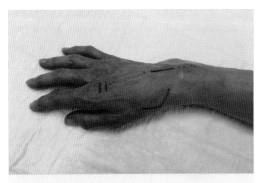

Fig. 9.3 Markings before extensor indicis transfer.

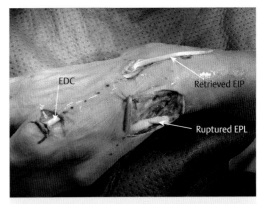

Fig. 9.4 Distal stump of extensor indicis is sutured to EDC over extensor zone 5 to reduce the risk of extensor lag in the index finger.

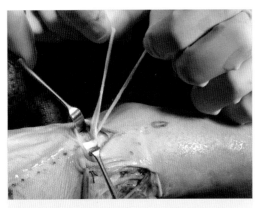

Fig. 9.5 EIP tendon is commonly found ulnar to the EDC tendon. In this case two slips of EIP were identified, which is present in 15% of cases.

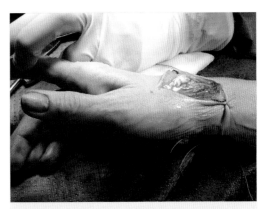

Fig. 9.6 EI tendon is weaved using the Pulvertaft technique to EPL using 3.0 Ethibond or PDS, with the wrist in neutral, it is tied to maximum tension to account for loosening in the postoperative period. The transfer is easier to adjust tension if done under local anesthetic and adrenaline.

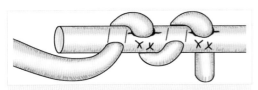

Fig. 9.7 Illustration of the Pulvertaft weave technique.

9.2 Rehabilitation after EIP to EPL Transfer

The patient is placed postoperatively in a forearm-based splint with the repair protected in a thumb spica extension cast. The plaster of Paris splint is changed to a thermoplastic splint on day 3 and early active mobilization is started. A protective splint must be worn for 12 weeks.

9.3 Closed Flexor Tendon Ruptures

The most likely closed tendon rupture to be encountered on a hand trauma list is an FDP avulsion. The classic presentation involves the ring finger of a young rugby player who has grabbed an opponent's shirt (jersey finger) avulsing the FDP from its insertion on the distal phalanx (▶ Fig. 9.8). Leddy and Packer classified these injuries into three types. In type 1, the tendon avulses from the distal phalanx and retracts to the palm, whereas in type 2, the intact vinculum longus limits retraction to the level of the proximal interphalangeal joint (PIPJ). Surgical repair of these injuries involves reinserting the FDP into the distal phalanx, which can be performed by a variety of techniques (pull-out sutures, transosseous sutures, Mitek mini anchors, etc.) (▶ Fig. 9.9, ▶ Fig. 9.10, ▶ Fig. 9.11, ▶ Fig. 9.12, ▶ Fig. 9.13). A type 3 avulsion involves a large bony fragment attached to the FDP tendon, which is held at the distal interphalangeal joint (DIPJ) by the A5 pulley (▶ Fig. 9.14). These injuries can be fixed either with screws, interosseous wire

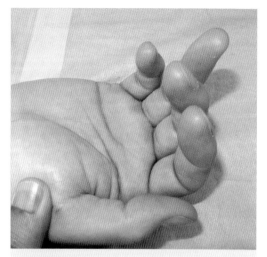

Fig. 9.8 Right ring finger closed FDP avulsion. Note the abnormal cascade.

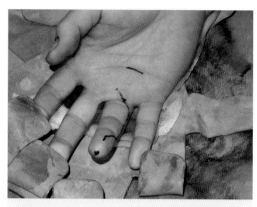

Fig. 9.9 Preoperative markings showing midlateral access to retrieve closed FDP rupture.

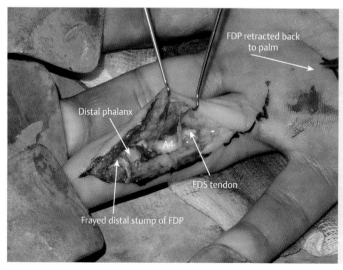

FDP retracted back to palm

Distal phalanx

A4

FDS tendon

Frayed distal stump of FDP

Fig. 9.10 FDP retracted back into the palm, frayed distal stump of FDP visible. Decision made to retrieve FDP from A1 pulley and preserve flexor sheath.

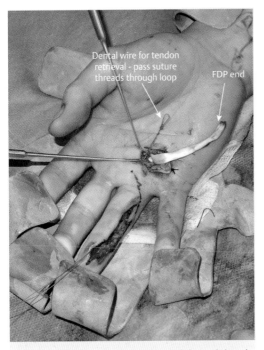

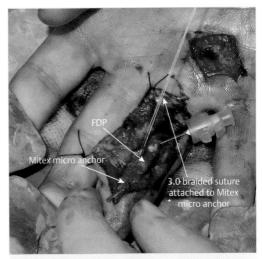

Fig. 9.12 Mitek micro anchor secured into distal phalanx. The whole hand should be raised off the arm table with the Mitek micro anchor to ensure that solid purchase has been made. Finally, repair of the proximal FDP stump to the Mitek micro anchor suture with a Bunnell-type repair.

Fig. 9.11 Retrieval of retracted FDP with looped dental wire. A suture is passed twice through the tip of the FDP to make it conical so that it can be easily passed through the pulleys. The suture is then passed through the dental wire loop.

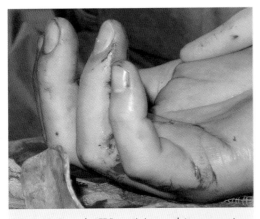

Fig. 9.13 Once the FDP repair is complete one must assess the tenodesis of the digit and ensure that the repair has been appropriately tightened.

fixation, or miniplate depending on the size of the bone fragment (▶ Fig. 9.15).

Occasionally, there can be an additional transverse fracture of the distal phalanx, which must also be fixed. This can be done either with an axial 1.1-mm K-wire, which often has to cross the DIPJ, combined with screw fixation of the fragment, or with a miniplate.

Closed tendon ruptures with less typical presentations should be carefully assessed and considered. Closed flexor tendon rupture after relatively trivial trauma, particularly in the older age group, may be due to attrition rupture at the wrist secondary to osteoarthritis or a prominent (volar) distal radial plate (▶ Fig. 9.16). These are seldom amenable to direct repair and require tendon reconstruction plus removal of the metalwork. An ultrasound can help determine the level of the tendon rupture, or least whether the tendon's distal insertion is intact.

Simultaneous loss of FDP index and FPL function without a history of trauma should make the surgeon consider anterior interosseous nerve syndrome. This is thought to be secondary to neuritis (a variant of Parsonage-Turner syndrome). Here, the tenodesis test will demonstrate tendon continuity,

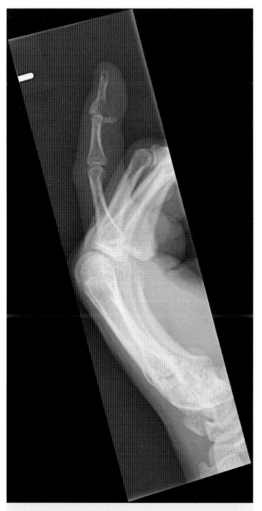

Fig. 9.14 Leddy Packer 3 FDP avulsion with large volar bone fragment.

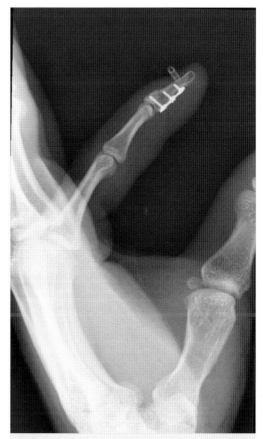

Fig. 9.15 Reduction of Leddy Packer 3 with miniplate.

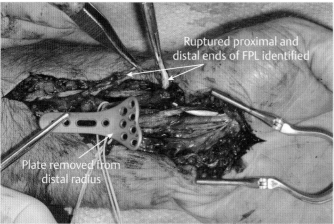

Ruptured proximal and distal ends of FPL identified

Plate removed from distal radius

Fig. 9.16 Flexor pollicis longus attrition rupture due to volar locking plate.

which can be confirmed on ultrasound. Nerve conduction studies will confirm the diagnosis. The initial management is conservative, with surgical decompression only in cases demonstrating no recovery at 6 months.

9.4 Rehabilitation after Repair of FDP Avulsion

Patients are seen with hand therapy in the first 3 days and are placed in a protective dorsal thermoplastic splint with the wrist in neutral and the metacarpophalangeal joint (MCPJ) in flexion at 70 degrees. Patients are all started on an early active mobilization regime and the splint should be worn continuously for 4 weeks. In the following 4 weeks, splints can be removed in the daytime but should be worn at night. All splintage is removed by 8 weeks; if a pullout suture has been used, this is normally removed at this point. Normal activities can be resumed at 12 weeks.

Selected Readings

Germann G, Wagner H, Blome-Eberwein S, Karle B, Wittemann M. Early dynamic motion versus postoperative immobilization in patients with extensor indicis proprius transfer to restore thumb extension: a prospective randomized study. J Hand Surg Am. 2001; 26(6):1111–1115

Prospective randomized trial comparing two rehabilitation protocols following EIP to EPL transfer: early dynamic motion and immobilization. The patients were assessed by measuring range of thumb motion, grip strength, and time needed off work. Patients who underwent immobilization were treated in a thumb spica splint for 3 weeks after surgery and the early mobilization group commenced gentle exercises on postoperative day 3. The results demonstrated improved range of motion at 3 weeks in patients assigned to the early dynamic motion protocol with similar findings noted when evaluating grip strength and pinch grip. However, at 6 and 8 weeks both groups had similar levels of function. The authors conclude that due to the fact that early mobilization allows for faster return of hand function and shortening of the rehabilitation time, it is a cost-effective solution and they recommend it as standard treatment for this patient population.

Gonzalez MH, Weinzweig N, Kay T, Grindel S. Anatomy of the extensor tendons to the index finger. J Hand Surg Am. 1996; 21(6):988–991

An anatomical study of 72 cadaveric specimens with the aim of delineating the course and the variations of the extensor tendons to the index finger. In 80% of cases, the tendons had a "classic" course

with a single extensor digitorum communis (EDC) and a single EIP tendon running to the index finger and the EIP assuming an ulnar position relative to the EDC at the level of the metacarpal head. Around 15% of cases had a double slip of the EIP. Two cases had an EIP, which was located either volar or radial to the EDC at the level of the metacarpal head. Two cases were found to have two slips of the EDC at the level of the metacarpal head.

Kang N, Pratt A, Burr N. Miniplate fixation for avulsion injuries of the flexor digitorum profundus insertion. J Hand Surg [Br]. 2003; 28(4):363–368

The authors describe the use of a miniplate with cortical screws in five cases of FDP avulsion with a bone fragment. Near-normal congruity was restored together with bony union in all cases. Surgery was carried out under ring block anesthesia. The fracture site was exposed with a midlateral incision. A 23-gauge needle was used to hold the FDP tendon out to length. A three- or two-hole miniplate was fashioned to conform the bone contour and then fixed with 1.5-mm screws. After tightening the screws, the fixation was checked by asking the patient to flex and extend under image intensifier.

Lalonde DH. Wide-awake extensor indicis proprius to extensor pollicis longus tendon transfer. J Hand Surg Am. 2014; 39(11):2297–2299

A description of performing the extensor indicis to extensor pollicis longus tendon transfer using wide-awake local anesthesia with no tourniquet. The patient undergoes injection of lidocaine with adrenaline into the subcutaneous plane at the operative site 30 minutes prior to commencing the procedure. The author argues that this translates to improved patient comfort, quicker discharge, and most importantly, it allows for the appropriate tensioning of the repair by asking the awake patient to move his or her thumb prior to skin closure to ensure that the repair is neither too tight or too loose.

Leddy JP, Packer JW. Avulsion of the profundus tendon insertion in athletes. J Hand Surg Am. 1977; 2(1):66–69

This seminal paper reviewed 36 avulsions of the flexor tendon insertion in athletes over 5 years in the ring finger. The authors classified the injuries based on three criteria: (1) presence or absence of bone fragment, (2) level of tendon retraction, and (3) status of blood supply of the avulsed tendon. The authors concluded that prompt surgical repair in these injuries gave the most optimal results.

Markeson DB, Mughal M, Subramanian P, Iyer S. The simple wire interosseous fixation technique (SWIFT) for reattachment of FDP avulsions with a large bony fragment. Tech Hand Up Extrem Surg. 2012; 16(4):220–224

In this technical paper, the authors describe the use of interosseous wire for FDP avulsions with a large bony fragment. Surgery is performed under local anesthesia and the approach is a volar Brunner incision centered over the DIPJ crease. The avulsion fracture is reduced with bone reduction forceps. Two white 19-gauge needles are passed through the avulsion bone fragment into the distal phalanx. A small incision in the dorsum of the digit allows the interosseous wire to loop around under the skin. The interosseous wire is then passed through the 19-gauge needles as a loop. The needles are then removed and the avulsion fragment is reduced by carefully tightening with wire loop.

10 Thumb MCP Joint Ulnar Collateral Ligament Repair

Dariush Nikkhah, Amir H. Sadr

Keywords: ulnar collateral ligament repair, Stener lesion, Skier thumb

10.1 Ulnar Collateral Ligament Repair

Acute rupture of the metacarpophalangeal joint (MCPJ) ulnar collateral ligament (UCL) also known as Skier thumb is a result of forced abduction that can further result in a UCL tear. The primary role

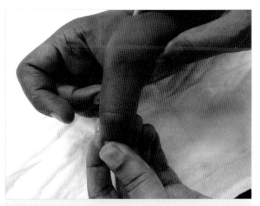

Fig. 10.1 Testing proper UCL in MCPJ flexion, no clear endpoint suggestive of UCL tear.

of the MCPJ of the thumb is flexion and extension. The joint is stabilized by the UCL and radial collateral ligament (RCL), the volar plate, and the dorsal capsule. The collateral ligaments consist of a strong proper collateral ligament and a weaker accessory collateral ligament.

To test for joint stability, one should test by fully flexing the MCPJ and should apply valgus stress to the thumb to test the proper collateral ligament. Laxity of over 35 degrees with no clear endpoint signifies rupture (▶ Fig. 10.1). Full extension of MCPJ with a valgus stress test assesses the accessory collateral ligament. One should make a comparison with the uninjured contralateral thumb.

If there is a midsubstance UCL rupture, a direct repair can be performed; however, in some cases Mitek mini anchor repair is warranted. The sequence of repair in both scenarios is illustrated in ▶ Fig. 10.2, ▶ Fig. 10.3, ▶ Fig. 10.4, ▶ Fig. 10.5, ▶ Fig. 10.6, ▶ Fig. 10.7, ▶ Fig. 10.8, ▶ Fig. 10.9, ▶ Fig. 10.10, ▶ Fig. 10.11, ▶ Fig. 10.12, ▶ Fig. 10.13, ▶ Fig. 10.14, ▶ Fig. 10.15, ▶ Fig. 10.16, ▶ Fig. 10.17, ▶ Fig. 10.18, ▶ Fig. 10.19. For an avulsion fracture of the UCL, one must assess the size of the bony fragment. If large, this can be fixed with a tension band K-wire technique (▶ Fig. 10.20).

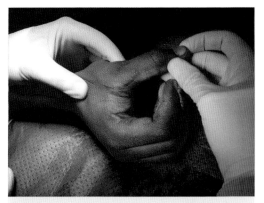

Fig. 10.2 A curvilinear incision is made over the UCL, making sure the incision is marked sufficiently volar to access the UCL.

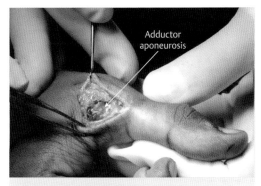

Fig. 10.3 After the skin incision, the adductor aponeurosis and hematoma are visualized; it is important not to divide the terminal branch of the superficial branch of radial nerve (SBRN) and retract it to one side.

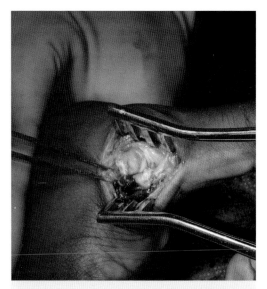

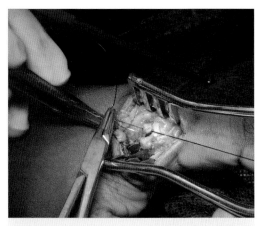

Fig. 10.5 As this is a midsubstance tear of the UCL, repair is achieved with a 3.0 PDS mattress suture. To provide additional strength, the dorsal joint capsule should also be repaired.

Fig. 10.4 Once the adductor aponeurosis is opened, access to UCL can be achieved. Here in the figure, the proximal end of the UCL is held with forceps.

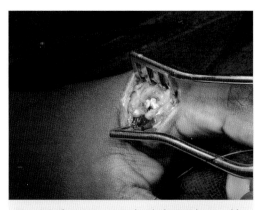

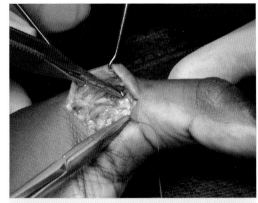

Fig. 10.6 The UCL is repaired with the PDS knot visible.

Fig. 10.7 Repair of the adductor aponeurosis with a 6.0 PDS running stitch.

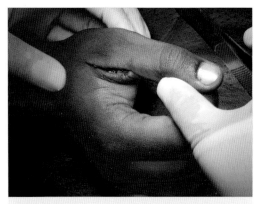

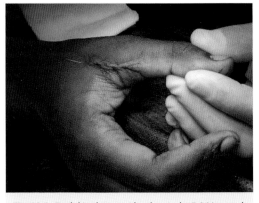

Fig. 10.8 After the final repair, the thumb is showing no laxity on valgus stress test.

Fig. 10.9 Final skin closure with subcuticular 5.0 Monocryl.

10.2 Stener Lesion

The entire UCL is normally covered by adductor aponeurosis. However, if the UCL is ruptured, its proximal end may be pulled out beneath the aponeurosis and become interposed between the adductor aponeurosis and its usual insertion point. This is a Stener lesion and can sometimes be palpated and is estimated to occur in half of UCL ruptures. Its importance is that the ligament will never heal due to it being interposed (▶ Fig. 10.10, ▶ Fig. 10.11, ▶ Fig. 10.12, ▶ Fig. 10.13, ▶ Fig. 10.14).

10.3 Rehabilitation after Ulnar Collateral Ligament Repair

The thumb should be placed in a thumb plaster of Paris cast immobilizing the MCPJ. This can be changed to a thumb spica splint which is worn full time for 4 to 6 weeks. The interphalangeal joint (IPJ) should be mobilized from the start and gentle MCPJ motion may start after 4 weeks if the pain has settled. Scar management is essential as the scar can become very tethered and sensitive.

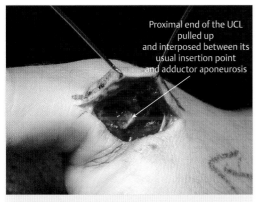

Proximal end of the UCL pulled up and interposed between its usual insertion point and adductor aponeurosis

Fig. 10.10 Stener lesion with proximal end of UCL visible over adductor aponeurosis.

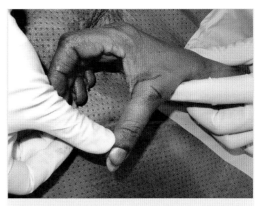

Fig. 10.11 Marked laxity of MCPJ suggestive of UCL rupture.

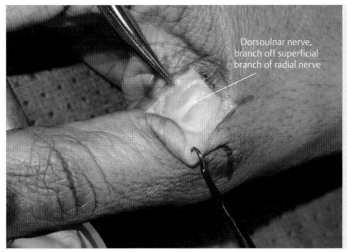

Dorsoulnar nerve, branch off superficial branch of radial nerve

Fig. 10.12 Terminal branch of SBRN identified and protected.

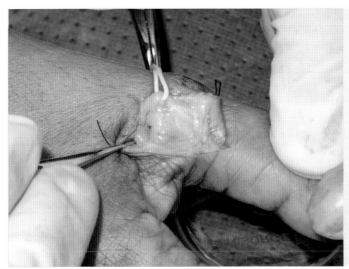

Fig. 10.13 Retraction of SBRN nerve, cut through adductor aponeurosis as marked in purple ink.

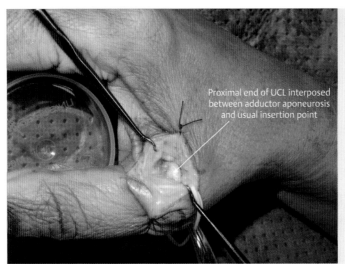

Proximal end of UCL interposed between adductor aponeurosis and usual insertion point

Fig. 10.14 Proximal end of UCL curled over adductor aponeurosis—so-called Stener lesion.

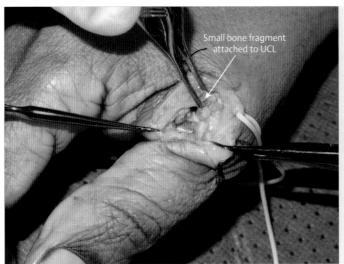

Small bone fragment attached to UCL

Fig. 10.15 Small bony segment avulsed off proximal phalanx, bony segment is removed before fixation with Mitek mini anchor onto the proximal phalanx.

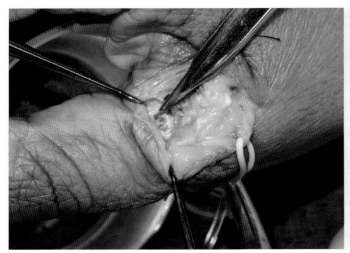

Fig. 10.16 Drill hole made in the proximal phalanx with white 18-gauge needle to accommodate Mitek mini anchor.

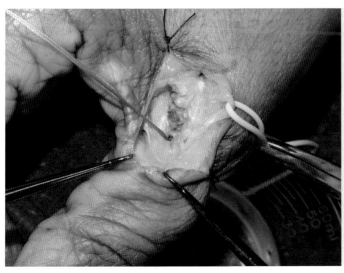

Fig. 10.17 Mitek mini anchor fitted into bone and 2.0 Ticron used to pass through UCL as a half-modified Kessler suture.

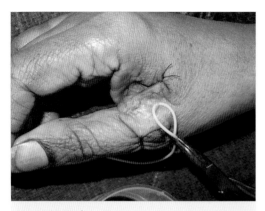

Fig. 10.18 Final repair.

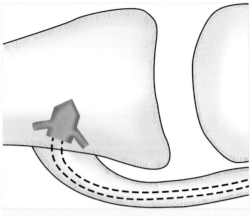

Fig. 10.19 Illustration of Mitek mini anchor.

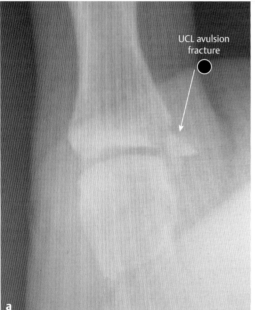

UCL avulsion
fracture

a

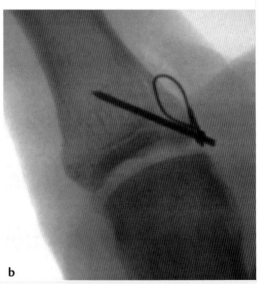

b

Fig. 10.20 (a,b) Tension band wire technique for UCL avulsion with large bony fragment.

Selected Readings

Campbell CS. Gamekeeper's thumb. J Bone Joint Surg Br. 1955; 37-B (1):148–149

Description of chronic repetitive injury as a nontraumatic cause for rupture of the UCL. The Scottish surgeon analyzed a total of 24 gamekeepers who killed rabbits by stretching and hyperextending the neck using their dominant hand. All cases of gamekeepers using this technique had demonstrable laxity of the UCL of the thumb, with the severity of damage found to be directly related to the number of rabbits terminated in this manner. Interestingly, despite positive examination findings, only a third of patients were symptomatic with the remaining 66% unaware of the presence of this pathology.

Hinke DH, Erickson SJ, Chamoy L, Timins ME. Ulnar collateral ligament of the thumb: MR findings in cadavers, volunteers, and patients with ligamentous injury (gamekeeper's thumb). AJR Am J Roentgenol. 1994; 163(6):1431–1434

Prospective study designed to determine the value of preoperative magnetic resonance imaging (MRI) in cases of suspected UCL tears. Eleven patients were included into the study and a separate anatomical study was performed on cadaveric specimens to establish the best method of imaging the ligament. Oblique/coronal T1 weighted was most useful for determining the anatomical details of the UCL. The MRI had 100% sensitivity for UCL injury; however, it was not accurate at determining the difference between simple tears and Stener's lesions. Out of three cases of surgically confirmed Stener's lesions, two were picked up by MRI, with further two cases of false-positive results.

Stener B. Displacement of the ruptured ulnar collateral ligament of the metacarpophalangeal joint. J Bone Joint Surg Am. 1962; 44B (4):869–879

A clinical and anatomical study conducted by Bertil Stener of Sweden in his seminal paper from 1962. A total of 40 cases were included into the description of this pathology, with over 80% of these being acute presentations and the remainder being chronically deficient in UCL function of the thumb. Stener also performed an anatomical investigation on a total of 42 postmortem specimens. The operative technique and the interposition of the adductor aponeurosis in between the two stumps of the ligament were described. The classic Stener's lesion has been noted to occur more commonly in distally ruptured ligaments (most common type) with displacement of the proximal stump in a position that is superficial in relation to the aponeurosis.

11 Digital Nerve Repair

Dariush Nikkhah

Keywords: digital nerve, epineural repair, nerve graft

11.1 Digital Nerve Repair

Digital nerve injuries are common in hand trauma and the most frequently injured are the peripheral nerves. Best outcomes in terms of sensory recovery are seen in children and young adults with more variable results in adults. The prime goals after epineural repair are to achieve some sensory recovery and to reduce the chances of neuroma formation. Digital nerve repair should ideally be done under a microscope to facilitate accurate epineural repair (▶ Fig. 11.1, ▶ Fig. 11.2, ▶ Fig. 11.3). In some cases, injury, secondary to machinery such as a powered circular saw, can result in segmental defects that cannot be repaired end to end. This necessitates nerve grafting either from the forearm or dorsal wrist. Other options include vein conduits, although these are only effective in short nerve gaps of 1 cm. If nerve gaps are greater than 1 cm, the vein conduit is likely to collapse, thereby impeding nerve regeneration.

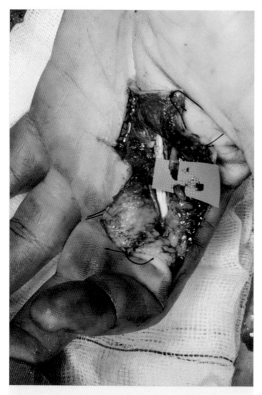

Fig. 11.1 Cut ends of radial digital nerve secondary to a knife laceration.

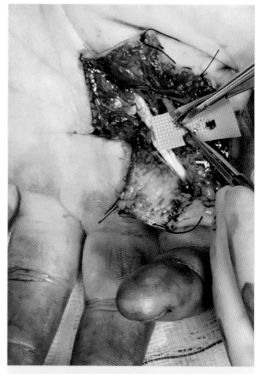

Fig. 11.2 Using a green background, the ends of the divided digital nerve are cut clean in preparation for epineural repair.

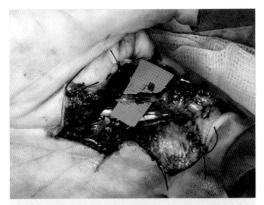

Fig. 11.3 Four 8.0 Ethilon stitches were used to repair the nerve. Usually the ends of the first two stitches are kept long so the surgeon can turn the repair around to do the back wall stitches.

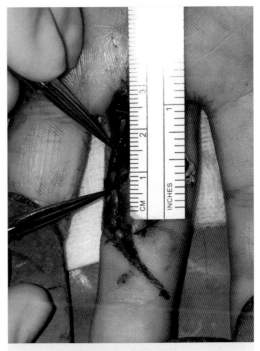

Fig. 11.4 Segmental nerve defect between jeweller's forceps secondary to circular saw.

11.2 Nerve Grafting for Segmental Defects

The case demonstrated highlights a segmental defect of 1 cm, which cannot be repaired primarily end to end (▶ Fig. 11.4). Many authors feel that nerve grafting is the gold standard approach for repair in these injuries. Donor site includes the forearm, either the medial or lateral antebrachial nerves of the forearm. These nerves run suprafascially and with the superficial veins (▶ Fig. 11.5, ▶ Fig. 11.6). The branches of the main nerves should be ideally taken to minimize donor site morbidity. The nerve stumps can also be buried into the muscle to reduce the risk of donor site neuroma. Finally, an end-to-end repair without tension is achieved with the nerve graft (▶ Fig. 11.7).

An alternative site for digital nerve graft harvest is the posterior interosseous nerve (PIN), which is located in the dorsal wrist (▶ Fig. 11.8).

11.3 Rehabilitation after Digital Nerve Repair

Digital nerve injuries distal to the metacarpophalangeal joint (MCPJ) are generally not splinted unless the repair is tight. All palmar and tight repairs have a splint for 2 weeks to limit the risk of damage. All patients start early motion, scar management as soon as possible, and sensory reeducation.

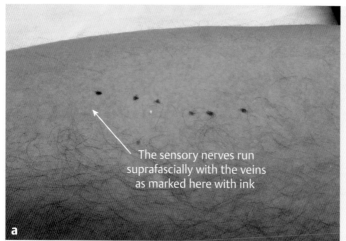

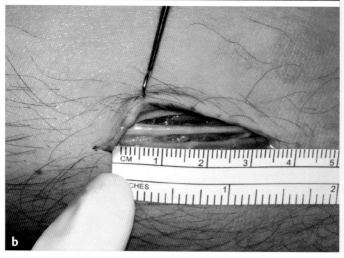

Fig. 11.5 (a,b) The nerve branches run with the veins above the fascia. The veins should be marked before the elevation of the tourniquet and thin skin flaps raised. The segment of donor nerve is measured for resection.

The sensory nerves run suprafascially with the veins as marked here with ink

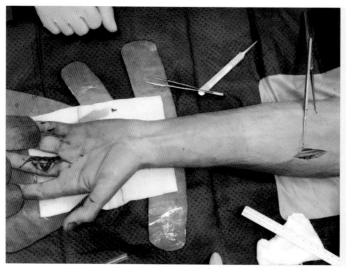

Fig. 11.6 Bird's eye view of donor site and recipient site for nerve graft.

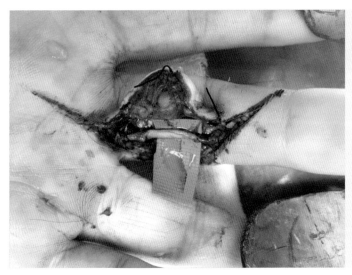

Fig. 11.7 The nerve is repaired end to end to the proximal and distal stumps of the recipient site with 8.0 Ethilon.

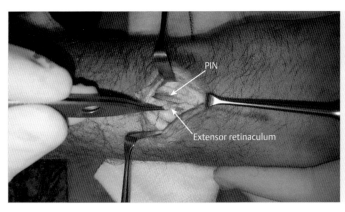

PIN

Extensor retinaculum

Fig. 11.8 One can harvest up to 3.5 cm of PIN graft material. This nerve is located under the extensor retinaculum on the radial aspect of the fourth extensor compartment.

Selected Readings

Clare TD, de Haviland Mee S, Belcher HJ. Rehabilitation of digital nerve repair: is splinting necessary? J Hand Surg [Br]. 2004; 29 (6):552–556

Study examining the effect of postoperative splinting on 40 sharp digital nerve lesions. No difference in sensibility between groups; however, the splinted group had a higher rate of stiffness and cold intolerance.

Fakin RM, Calcagni M, Klein HJ, Giovanoli P. Long-term clinical outcome after epineural coaptation of digital nerves. J Hand Surg Eur Vol. 2016; 41(2):148–154

Prospective cohort study to determine clinical outcomes in adults undergoing epineural end-to-end digital nerve repair. Mean follow-up was 3.5 years with all patients being evaluated for sensory recovery using two-point discrimination and Semmes-Weinstein monofilament testing. A total of 93 repaired digital nerves were included into the study, with symptomatic neuroma formation being seen in two cases. No patient recovered functional sensibility; however, protective sensation was present in all cases and this was found to be an important factor determining patient satisfaction with surgical intervention. Mean 2PD was 10.6 mm and mean Semmes-Weinstein monofilament value was 2.7 (2.2 on contralateral side). The only preoperative predictor of sensory outcome was the experience of the operating surgeon.

Slutsky DJ. The management of digital nerve injuries. J Hand Surg Am. 2014; 39(6):1208–1215

Review paper evaluating the immediate management and long-term outcomes of digital nerve repair. Primary end-to-end neurorrhaphy is recommended when dealing with clean lacerations of the nerve and where the stumps can be mobilized to adjoin without tension. Specific techniques of primary nerve repair did not significantly differ in terms of sensory recovery. Younger age was found to be associated with improved outcomes. Where the stumps have formed a gap of 4 mm or more, the use of autologous nerve graft or conduit has superior results to primary repair. Delay in nerve repair was not found to be related to long-term sensory recovery.

Thomas PR, Saunders RJ, Means KR. Comparison of digital nerve sensory recovery after repair using loupe or operating microscope magnification. J Hand Surg Eur Vol. 2015; 40(6):608–613

Study evaluating the clinical outcomes following digital nerve repair using epineural coaptation with loupe magnification versus operating microscope. A total of 13 digital nerves were repaired using loupe magnification and 12 nerves repaired under the operating microscope. The patients were followed up for a period of 24 months by a therapist who was blinded to the operative approach. There were no significant differences when evaluating static and moving two-point discrimination or Semmes-Weinstein monofilament testing. The authors recommend that as long as one is adequately trained in the principles of nerve repair, loupe magnification is sufficient to achieve satisfactory outcomes.

12 Replantation and Revascularization

Dariush Nikkhah

Keywords: replantation, revascularization, vein graft

12.1 Thumb Revascularization with Vein Graft

The thumb constitutes 40% of hand function and attempt for salvage must be always made. However, it poses a challenge in terms of microsurgical access and positioning. The ulnar digital artery (UDA) is dominant compared to the radial digital artery (RDA) and there is often a good dorsal supply in the thumb from the princeps pollicis artery. If there is complete division of the UDA and RDA, the thumb can sometimes maintain sufficient vascularity with the dorsal supply.

In both thumb revascularization and replantation, vein grafting is usually required as tensionless anastomosis of the arteries is rarely possible. Jump vein grafting out of the zone of trauma to the radial artery in the anatomical snuff box enables a reliable anastomosis and avoids the technical difficulties of thumb positioning during microsurgery. We describe the sequence of steps in a case where a thumb was revascularized after a circular saw injury at the level of the interphalangeal joint (IPJ) (▶ Fig. 12.1, ▶ Fig. 12.2, ▶ Fig. 12.3, ▶ Fig. 12.4, ▶ Fig. 12.5, ▶ Fig. 12.6, ▶ Fig. 12.7).

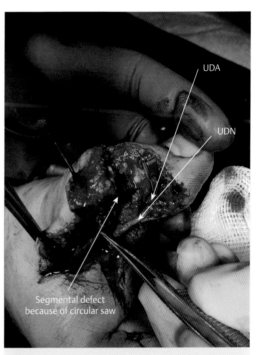

Fig. 12.2 Both the volar neurovascular structures are divided in this case with a segmental defect. The UDA is identified distally and resected to healthy artery just proximal to the trifurcation. The UDA cannot be identified proximally in this figure. A single Acland's clamp is placed over the distal UDA. UDA, ulnar digital artery; UDN, ulnar digital nerve.

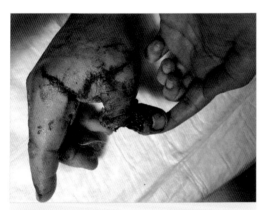

Fig. 12.1 Circular saw injury through thumb IPJ. Thumb held on by small dorsal skin bridge and the FPL tendon. Capillary refill is not present and oxygen saturations reading is unrecordable.

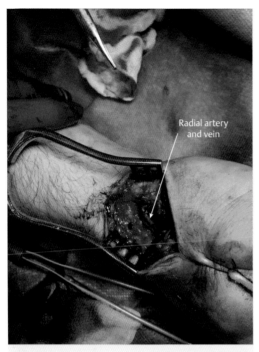

Fig. 12.3 Radial artery identified in the anatomical snuff box.

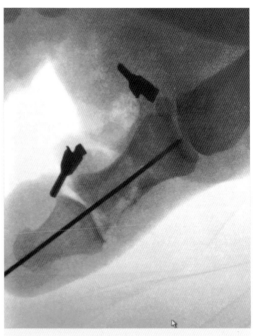

Fig. 12.4 Rapid osteosynthesis performed with single axial K-wire passed retrograde first before driving wire across IPJ.

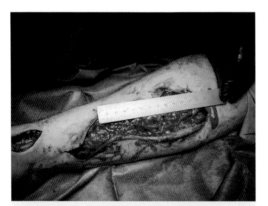

Fig. 12.5 Because of the large zone of injury and poor flow from the proximal cut end of UDA and princeps pollicis artery. A jump vein graft was harvested from the forearm.

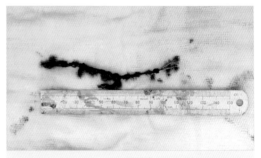

Fig. 12.6 An 11-cm vein graft was taken from the forearm. An alternative site can be the vena comitans of the radial artery in the wrist. Plenty of fat was taken to cushion the vein graft and allow for swifter harvest. Ink and an Acland clamp mark the proximal extent of the vein as it needs to be turned around due to valves.

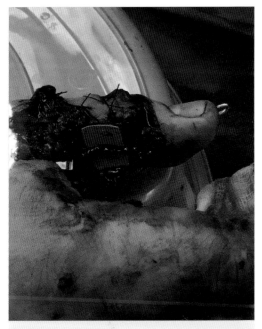

Fig. 12.7 The harvested vein graft was bridged from the radial artery to the UDA. A double Acland clamp isolated a segment of the radial artery in the snuff box and an end-to-side anastomosis was performed with 9.0 ST. The distal anastomosis was performed end to end with the UDA.

12.2 Digital Replantation

Digital replantation follows a sequence of steps and can be performed if the principles in the previous chapters in this book are learned (▶ Fig. 12.8, ▶ Fig. 12.9, ▶ Fig. 12.10, ▶ Fig. 12.11, ▶ Fig. 12.12, ▶ Fig. 12.13, ▶ Fig. 12.14, ▶ Fig. 12.15, ▶ Fig. 12.16, ▶ Fig. 12.17, ▶ Fig. 12.18, ▶ Fig. 12.19, ▶ Fig. 12.20, ▶ Fig. 12.21, ▶ Fig. 12.22, ▶ Fig. 12.23, ▶ Fig. 12.24, ▶ Fig. 12.25, ▶ Fig. 12.26, ▶ Fig. 12.27, ▶ Fig. 12.28, ▶ Fig. 12.29). Osteosynthesis should be performed first to provide a stable platform followed by repair of macroscopic structures (tendons). Microscopic structures should then be repaired (nerve, artery, veins). Amputations of the thumb, pediatric amputation, and multidigit loss are all absolute indications for replantation. However, some cases where there are crush or avulsion injuries, success rates are poor and in the figure of 50 to 60%. Success does not just rely on survival but on long-term function and replantation proximal to the flexor digitorum superficialis (FDS) insertion may never regain a normal range of motion.

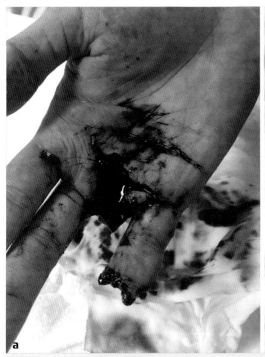

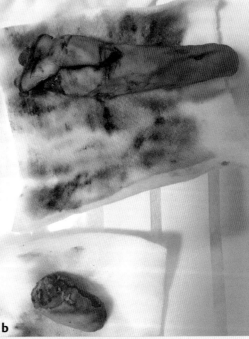

a   b

Fig. 12.8 (a,b) Avulsion crush amputation of little and ring fingers. Digits were wrapped in wet gauze in a plastic bag placed on ice. The amputated part should never be placed directly on ice.

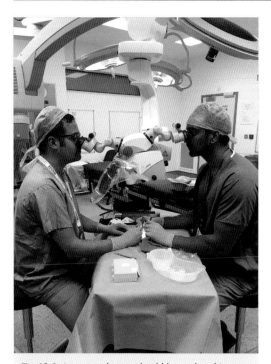

Generally, clean-cut amputations distal to the FDS insertion with minimal ischemic time (< 12 hours warm ischemia) do well. Those with avulsion-type mechanism and long ischemic time have poorer outcomes as in the case demonstrated; and in many cases a no-reflow phenomenon occurs. Patient selection is therefore crucial and if an anastomosis is to be performed in a crush avulsion case, it should be done outside of a zone of trauma and in some cases vein grafts may be necessary to increase the chances of success.

Fig. 12.9 Amputated parts should be explored in theater to see if there are any suitable vessels. This will buy time while the patient is being anesthetized. The amputated digit can be stabilized during this process with pins and vascular loops. In a multidigit amputation, if one amputated part is unreplantable it should be used for "spare parts" for the remaining digits.

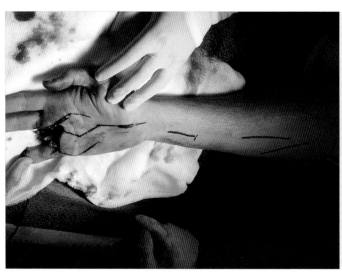

Fig. 12.10 Vein grafts marked in proximal forearm before arm exsanguination.

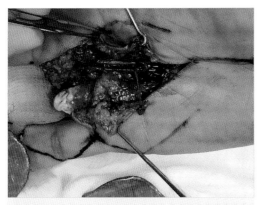

Fig. 12.11 Common digital nerve and artery found outside zone of trauma proximally.

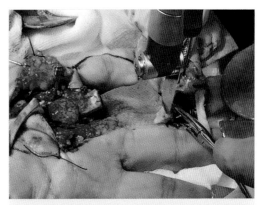

Fig. 12.12 Bone ends are shortened in preparation for osteosynthesis. Glove used to protect neurovascular bundles.

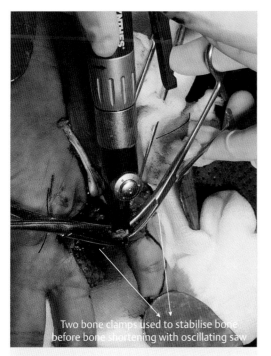

Two bone clamps used to stabilise bone before bone shortening with oscillating saw

Fig. 12.13 Cross-clamping method to stabilize bone before shortening.

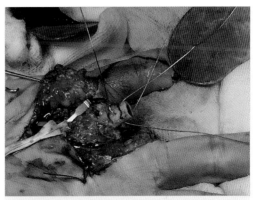

Fig. 12.14 90–90 wiring used to bring bone ends together rapidly. This avoids the use of a C-arm during the procedure and is rapid, cheap, and provides excellent bone-to-bone contact.

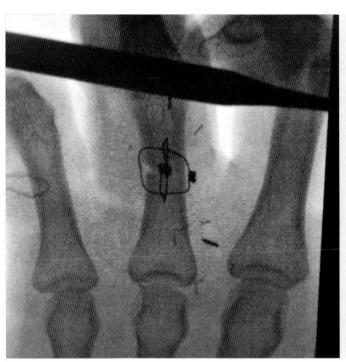

Fig. 12.15 Radiograph of box wires.

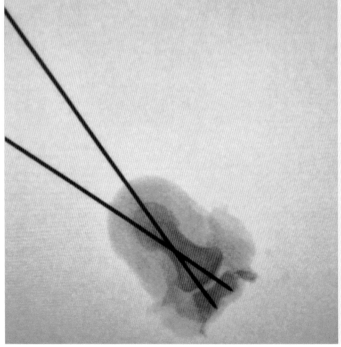

Fig. 12.16 Alternative method of fixation is K-wires. Amputated part is prepared first with retrograde pass of two 0.9 K-wires.

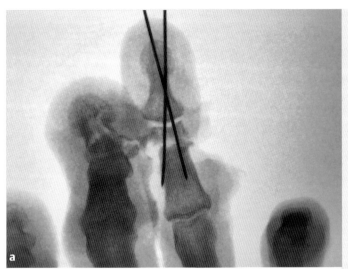

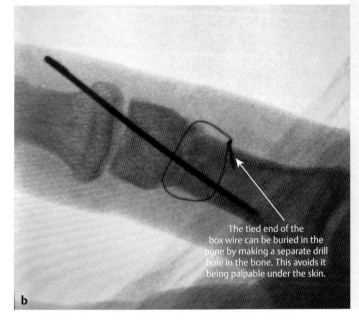

Fig. 12.17 (a,b) Alternative methods of osteosynthesis include retrograde cross K-wire fixation or a single K-wire and a loop of interosseous wire described by Lister.

The tied end of the box wire can be buried in the bone by making a separate drill hole in the bone. This avoids it being palpable under the skin.

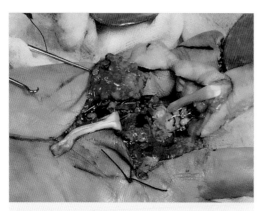

Fig. 12.18 Completed intraoperative 90–90 box wiring.

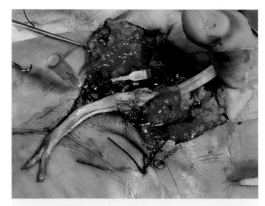

Fig. 12.19 Next the flexor digitorum profundus (FDP) tendon is repaired with preservation of the A2 pulley. The FDS was not repaired as it had been avulsed from the bone and FDS repair would compromise tendon glide. The extensor tendon is next repaired.

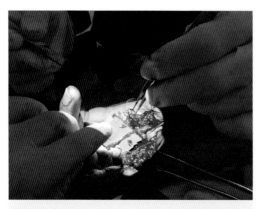

Fig. 12.20 Nerve repair is performed next under tourniquet. If nerves cannot be repaired, then the digit will have no use as an insensate digit. The tourniquet is then let down and arterial anastomosis is performed. One must check that there is good flow proximally by releasing the Acland clamp.

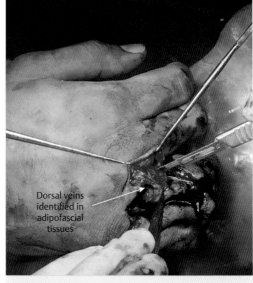

Dorsal veins identified in adipofascial tissues

Fig. 12.21 Veins can be difficult to find and can be easily found in the adipofascial tissue under the dorsal skin flaps. After arterial anastomosis, they become engorged and more readily visible. Ideally, two venous anastomoses should be performed.

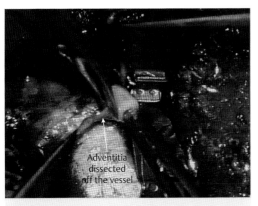

Fig. 12.22 When preparing for the arterial anastomosis, the adventitia is stripped off. The artery is then dilated with vessel dilators.

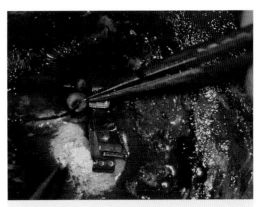

Fig. 12.23 Heparin saline is used to irrigate the vessel lumen and remove any visible clots.

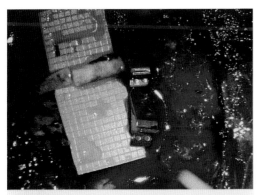

Fig. 12.24 The artery is prepared for anastomosis. A single Acland clamp can be used and a background helps with visualization.

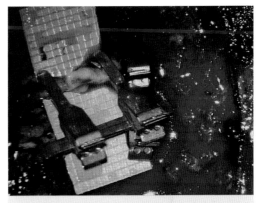

Fig. 12.25 A double Acland provides more optimal control and enables the repair of the anterior wall first and then turning over for posterior wall repair. This is, however, not always possible in a confined space and a back wall first anastomosis must be performed.

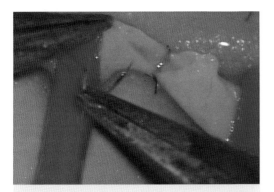

Fig. 12.26 The best way to avoid catching the posterior wall with anterior wall stitches is to suture the back wall first.

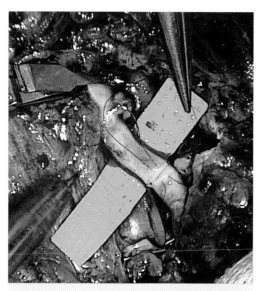

Fig. 12.27 The final stitches on the anterior wall are done using an untied Harashina stitch. This reduces the chances of catching the back wall of the anastomosis.

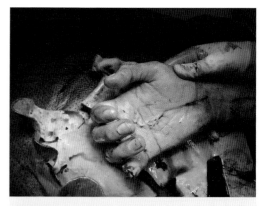

Fig. 12.28 Completed replantation of ring finger.

12.3 Postoperative Management in Replantation

Venous congestion is the most common postoperative complication seen in digital replantation. Ideally, as many veins as possible should be anastomosed. If congestion does occur, options include removing the nail plate, and scraping part of the nailbed to allow for bleeding with heparin-soaked gauze. An alternative method is to use leeches. Reexploration with reanastomoses of the veins can be challenging and often unsuccessful.

The color, turgor, and capillary refill of the replanted digit should be assessed and if there is difficulty particularly in the darker-skinned patient, a pulse oximeter probe can be used for an objective assessment.

12.4 Rehabilitation after Digital Replantation

The replanted digit and hand are protected in a volar splint in the position of safe immobilization for the first week. The original splint fashioned in theater is usually changed on day 3 for a thermoplastic splint. Care must be taken when changing the dressing not to compress the replanted digit. Early active range of motion can be started as soon as the vascularity is stable. This is important especially if a plate fixation is used. For Kirschner wire, fixation exercises should be started to the joints not immobilized with the wires.

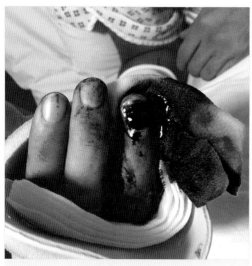

Fig. 12.29 Congested digit managed with heparin-soaked gauze to allow bleeding from the nailbed.

Selected Readings

Barbary S, Dap F, Dautel G. Finger replantation: surgical technique and indications. Chir Main. 2013; 32(6):363–372

Review article of the surgical techniques of digital replantation, with particular focus on replantation of the thumb, pediatric fingertips, distal replants, and ring avulsion injuries. Principles of meticulous surgical technique, adequate debridement, and systematized approach to repair are highlighted. Indications for replantation listed by the authors include thumb amputations, multiple digit amputations, pediatric amputations, amputations distal to the FDS insertion, and transmetacarpal or more proximal amputations.

Breahna A, Siddiqui A, Fitzgerald O'Connor E, Iwuagwu FC. Replantation of digits: a review of predictive factors for survival. J Hand Surg Eur Vol. 2016; 41(7):753–757

Retrospective analysis of a single regional unit experience of digital replantation in a 4-year period. About 75 cases were included into the study and the demographics, medical histories, and postoperative outcome were reviewed. Survival rate of 70% was seen with arterial thrombosis being the leading cause of replantation failure. Multivariate analysis demonstrated association of warm ischemic time less than 6 hours and 30 minutes and replantations done within "office hours" with improved rates of survival of replanted digits.

Harashina T. Use of the united suture in microvascular anastomoses. Plast Reconstr Surg. 1977; 59(1):134–135

Technical paper describing the use of an untied suture as the last suture in the anastomoses. This avoids picking up the posterior wall with the anterior wall.

Morrison WA, McCombe D. Digital replantation. Hand Clin. 2007; 23(1):1–12

Review paper evaluating optimal management of digital replantation. Incomplete amputations of the digit have an increased chance of successful replantation when compared to complete amputation. Guillotine mechanism of injury is also favorable in these cases.

Decision to replant a digit should be made by weighing up the potential contribution the digit can make to hand function versus probability that it may in fact reduce remaining hand function. Warm ischemic time of less than 12 hours and cold ischemic time of less than 24 hours are associated with higher rates of successful replantation. Operative technique relies on prompt identification of all vital structures at the amputation site and severed stump followed by debridement of nonviable tissue. Bone shortening and fixation is performed first, followed by flexor and extensor tendon repair, neurorrhaphy, and arterial and venous anastomoses. Lastly, the skin and soft-tissue envelope is closed. Meticulous operative technique in tendon repair is essential to allow for early movement and ultimately a good functional outcome.

Nikkhah D, Sadr AH, Murugesan L, Konczalik W, Rodrigues J. Cross-clamping of bony stumps in preparation for osteosynthesis in digital replantation. Microsurgery. 2017; 37(4):356–357

Technical paper describing an effective method of stabilization of bony stumps prior to debridement with the osteotome. Adequate shortening of the bone is imperative to obtain stable fixation and ultimately a good functional outcome of the digit. Application of two artery forceps to the stump will allow for the surgeon to gain better control of the stump and achieve a more precise cut. By wrapping a glove around the neurovascular bundles one can also minimize the risk to adjacent structures.

Shafiroff BB, Palmer AK. Simplified technique for replantation of the thumb. J Hand Surg Am. 1981; 6(6):623–624

A technical paper describing the use of jump vein grafting in thumb digital artery anastomoses. The author states that a reversed vein graft taken from the ipsilateral forearm/wrist can be anastomosed to the digital vessels prior to osteosynthesis. By doing so, one can avoid difficulties with the anastomosis resulting from positioning problems. This technique also proves useful when faced with large gaps between the vessel stumps that would not allow for tension-free repair.

13 The Spaghetti Wrist

Dariush Nikkhah, Wojciech Konczalik

Keywords: spaghetti wrist, nerve repair

13.1 Spaghetti Wrist

The spaghetti wrist can involve division of up to 16 structures (▶ Fig. 13.1). These injuries are commonly secondary to glass or knife lacerations and also to deliberate self-harm. A systematic approach is needed to avoid secondary complications and to optimize the efficiency of surgical repair (▶ Fig. 13.2, ▶ Fig. 13.3, ▶ Fig. 13.4, ▶ Fig. 13.5, ▶ Fig. 13.6, ▶ Fig. 13.7, ▶ Fig. 13.8, ▶ Fig. 13.9, ▶ Fig. 13.10, ▶ Fig. 13.11, ▶ Fig. 13.12, ▶ Fig. 13.13).

Glass injuries are often more extensive than you think. One must perform a detailed preoperative examination so that you can identify which structures are likely to be damaged and which ones you must identify. One should start the dissection outside the zone of trauma to help identify *normal* anatomy, and then follow normal structures into the zone of trauma. This avoids ineffective dissection around the wound.

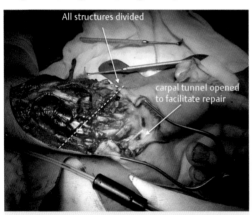

Fig. 13.1 Glass laceration to distal forearm with division of all structures including radial and ulnar arteries, the carpal tunnel has been opened to facilitate repair.

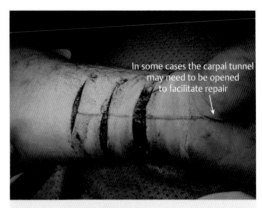

Fig. 13.2 Broad flaps should be designed and flaps should be taken with fascia to minimize flap necrosis. The carpal tunnel may need to be opened to facilitate repair and should be marked.

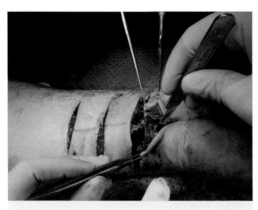

Fig. 13.3 Flaps being raised with fascia.

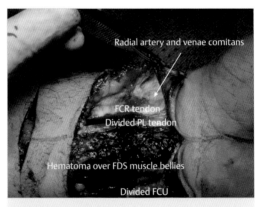

Fig. 13.4 Dissection should be systematic and should start with the radial or ulnar side of the wrist with a systematic assessment identifying damaged structures. Here you can see the radial artery and flexor carpi radialis (FCR) are intact.

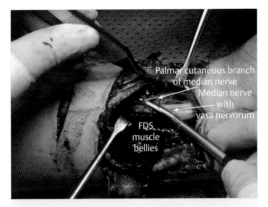

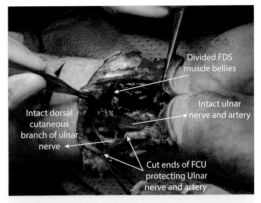

Fig. 13.5 The median nerve is identified under the divided palmaris longus and its palmar cutaneous branch is also identified.

Fig. 13.6 The figure shows the divided FDS muscle bellies and the FCU. The ulnar nerve and artery are not divided and were protected by the FCU tendon. The figure also shows the dorsal sensory branch of ulnar nerve.

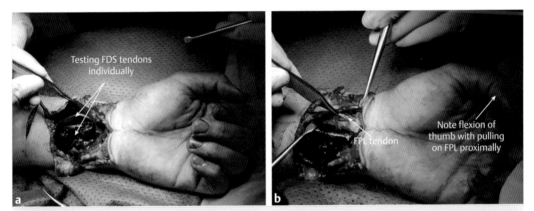

Fig. 13.7 **(a)** The FDS ring and the little finger are divided. The tendons are lifted to check each one individually. The FDS tendons to the ring and middle fingers are superficial to the index and small fingers. **(b)** The flexor pollicis longus (FPL) is the most radial structure in wrist and found to be intact if thumb flexion is present.

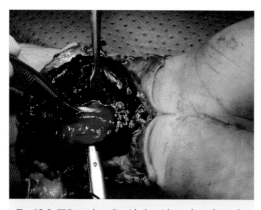

Fig. 13.8 FDP tendons lie side by side and are brought up and found to be intact.

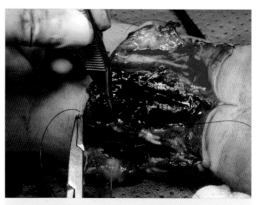

Fig. 13.9 Repair of the FCU is with a four-strand modified Kessler 3.0 Prolene; note flexion of the wrist will help accommodate the repair. If the FCU has retracted back, a back wall 5.0 epitendinous stitch will help draw the tendon ends together making the core stitch easier.

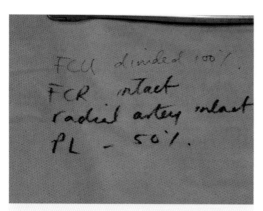

Fig. 13.10 Documentation of divided structures; important for the primary surgeon to keep track to prevent structures being missed.

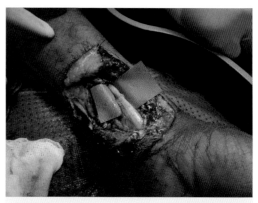

Fig. 13.11 Another case demonstrating completed median nerve repair with microscope using 8.0 Ethilon. The repair is epineural and the vasa nervorum have been used to align the nerve.

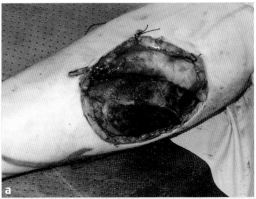
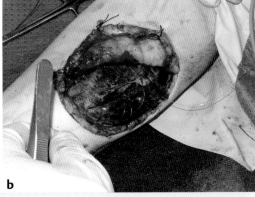

Fig. 13.12 (a,b) Many surgeons use Vicryl to repair muscle bellies. However, using Monocryl has certain advantages; as it is monofilament, it glides easily and multiple continuous loops, as in the figures, bring the muscles together without difficulty.

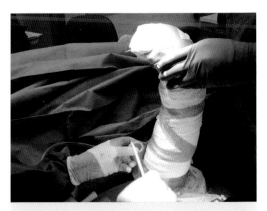

Fig. 13.13 Dorsal blocking splint to protect nerve and tendon repairs. Ensure the splint is securely taped on, so that it can last until it is changed for a thermoplastic splint.

13.2 Systematic Approach to Repair

During the spaghetti wrist repair, it is important to make note on the scrub table of the structures divided and tick them off once repaired. This will prevent confusion during long periods of surgery.

If the tourniquet time permits, repair the peripheral nerves without letting the tourniquet down. Use the vasa nervorum as a guide of where to orientate the nerve repair precisely. It is best to do the 12 and 6 o'clock repairs in a bivalve fashion and leave the threads of the 8.0 microsuture long to help facilitate turnover of the nerve for back wall epineural repair.

Arterial repair is best done when the tourniquet is down. The hand can still be vascularized from the posterior interosseous artery if both vessels are divided. Proximal dissection of the vessels can allow for a tensionless repair if the repair is tight. If there is a large segmental gap, the venae comitantes should be used as a bridging vein graft. A double Acland clamp provides good control and anastomosis is best performed with a back wall first technique.

13.3 Rehabilitation after Spaghetti Wrist

Patients are placed in a dorsal plaster of Paris splint after the surgery to protect the nerve and tendon repairs. Early active mobilization is started on day 3 to 5. These patients will require extensive hand therapy for many months: firstly, to protect the tendons, reduce the scar tissue, and tendon adherence in zone 5, and secondly to encourage nerve regeneration and improve hand function.

Selected Readings

Hudson DA, de Jager LT. The spaghetti wrist. Simultaneous laceration of the median and ulnar nerves with flexor tendons at the wrist. J Hand Surg [Br]. 1993; 18(2):171–173

   A prospective analysis of 15 patients sustaining lacerations to flexor zone 5 with damage to both median and ulnar nerves. Increasing numbers of flexor tendons involved was thought to be associated with poor outcomes. Out of a total of 76 tendons repaired in this case series, functional outcomes were excellent in almost half of the repairs; however, 20% were classified as fair and 25% of the cases were deemed functionally poor. Primary nerve repair allowed for return of protective sensation, with better recovery noted in median nerve lacerations than ulnar nerve lesions.

Jaquet JB, van der Jagt I, Kuypers PD, Schreuders TA, Kalmijn AR, Hovius SE. Spaghetti wrist trauma: functional recovery, return to work, and psychological effects. Plast Reconstr Surg. 2005; 115(6):1609–1617

   A retrospective single-center study of 67 spaghetti wrist injuries with a mean follow-up of 10 years. One-fourth of all cases were anesthetic on Semmes-Weinstein testing and the remainder only had recovery of protective sensation. All but two patients had functional disability as evidenced by the Functional Symptom Score. Almost 50% of all patients could not return to their job following their injury. Of those that did, the average time taken off work was 34 weeks. Evidence of psychological disturbance was present in two-thirds of patients during the first month following surgery.

Weinzweig N, Chin G, Mead M, Gonzalez M. "Spaghetti wrist": management and results. Plast Reconstr Surg. 1998; 102(1):96–102

   Retrospective analysis of 60 patients in a single center over a period of 8 years. Over two-thirds of the patients were males with an average age of 29 years. Accidental glass and knife lacerations constituted over 80% of all cases. The most commonly injured structures were the flexor carpi ulnaris (FCU), median nerve, flexor digitorum superficialis (FDS), and ulnar neurovascular bundle. The ulnar aspect of the wrist (FCU, ulnar vessels, and nerve) was more frequently involved than the radial or central aspect of the wrist. Only 30% of patients were followed up, and of these, range of motion was deemed excellent or good in all of cases; however, intrinsic muscle recovery was deemed fair to poor in over 40% of these cases.

14 Fracture Fixation Techniques

Dariush Nikkhah, Nikki Burr, Robert Pearl

Keywords: hand fractures, plate fixation, Kirschner wire fixation, external fixation

14.1 Jahss Maneuver

This is a useful technique to help manipulate the neck of fifth metacarpal fractures. It is also useful intraoperatively when fixing fifth metacarpal fractures. The fracture is reduced by flexing the metacarpophalangeal joint (MCPJ) and proximal interphalangeal joint (PIPJ) of the little finger to 90 degrees and using the proximal phalanx to push up the head of the fifth metacarpal thereby reducing it (▶ Fig. 14.1, ▶ Fig. 14.2, ▶ Fig. 14.3).

14.2 Salter-Harris 2 Fractures of the Proximal Phalanx

The most common type of Salter-Harris fracture involves fracture through the metaphysis of the proximal phalanx and it has an incidence of 80% (▶ Fig. 14.4). These injuries are very common in the emergency department and can easily be reduced using a pen as a fulcrum (▶ Fig. 14.5).

In older children, this manipulation can be done under local anesthetic and checked with fluoroscopic scan; otherwise, general anesthesia is needed. After reduction, the adjacent finger is buddy strapped to the injured finger and the hand

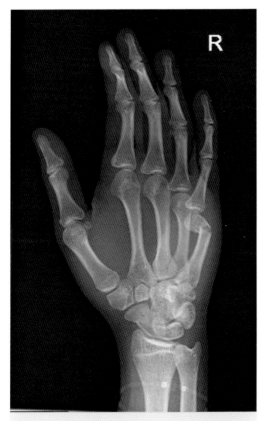

Fig. 14.1 Neck of the right fifth metacarpal fracture.

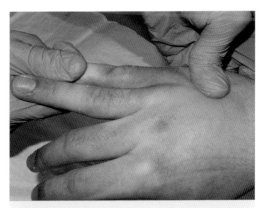

Fig. 14.2 Traction of fifth metacarpal fracture.

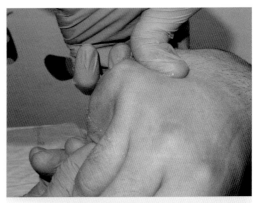

Fig. 14.3 Using proximal phalanx to push up the head of the fifth metacarpal while flexing the MCPJ and PIPJ (Jahss maneuver).

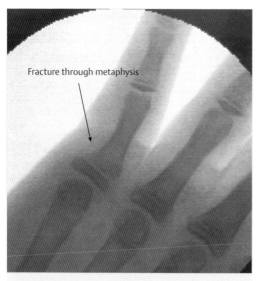

Fracture through metaphysis

Fig. 14.4 Radiograph of Salter-Harris 2 fracture of proximal phalanx of the little finger.

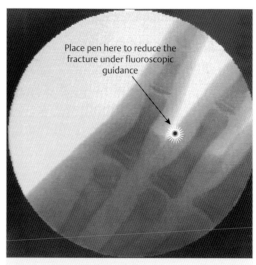

Place pen here to reduce the fracture under fluoroscopic guidance

Fig. 14.5 Postreduction in the same patient with a pen used as a fulcrum.

is rested in a volar splint before active mobilization at 1 week.

14.3 Conservative Management of Fractures

Hand surgeons, young and old, like to fix fractures. However, it is important to be selective and to identify cases where nonoperative management may be preferable (▶ Fig. 14.6). Many hand fractures can be treated conservatively as long as the fracture is stable, minimally displaced with no rotation or scissoring.

Placing metal work can interfere with tendon glide and these patients may need further surgery to remove the plate with the need for extensor tenolysis. The aim of all fracture fixations is a solid fixation so that early hand therapy can commence. It is no longer acceptable to keep patients in a plaster of Paris for 3 to 4 weeks postoperation.

14.3.1 Rehabilitation after Conservative Management

Patients are placed in a volar resting splint after assessment or fracture reduction. Early referral to the hand therapy team for education, protection of the fracture as necessary, and early edema control

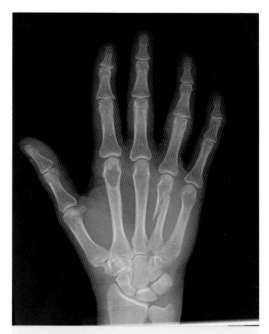

Fig. 14.6 The fourth metacarpal fracture managed conservatively. The fourth metacarpal unlike the fifth and second metacarpal is stabilized by the deep transverse metacarpal ligament on both sides, which runs across the palmar surfaces of the heads of the metacarpals.

is important. If there are any concerns regarding stability, a repeat radiograph at 1 week will confirm if the reduction of the fracture has been maintained. Early motion is essential for all stable fractures to prevent stiffness.

14.4 Kirschner Wire Fixation

Percutaneous K-wire fixation should be considered in many closed hand fracture configurations, where a satisfactory closed reduction has been achieved, but is unlikely to be maintained with splints or casts alone (▶ Fig. 14.7). However, K-wiring is not always easy to perform and sometimes multiple passes are made in error. To minimize problems, a number of simple steps can be performed.

One must mark the joints with a pen to help with the 3D understanding of the fracture. Radiologic markers such as a 25-gauge orange needle can help guide the trajectory of the K-wire (▶ Fig. 14.8, ▶ Fig. 14.9). However, when passing the K-wire one should go by *feeling* the resistance of the cortical bone. Furthermore, making small stab incisions through the skin with a 15 blade is useful rather than stabbing the K-wire through the skin inadvertently catching the extensor mechanism. If repeated attempts are made during surgery, a new K-wire should be loaded on the driver. Repeated attempts and high revolutions should be avoided as thermal damage to bone can result in problems with union and infection.

14.4.1 Rehabilitation after Kirschner Wire Fixation

The fracture is protected postsurgery in a volar plaster of Paris cast, which is replaced with a smaller splint after referral to hand therapy. Gentle active range-of-motion exercises are generally started after 1 week. The K-wire is removed at 3 to 4 weeks when fracture tenderness has reduced.

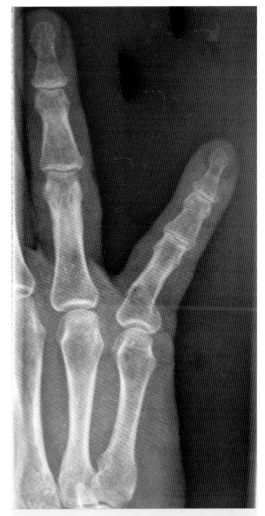

Fig. 14.7 Closed little finger proximal phalanx fracture with significant angulation.

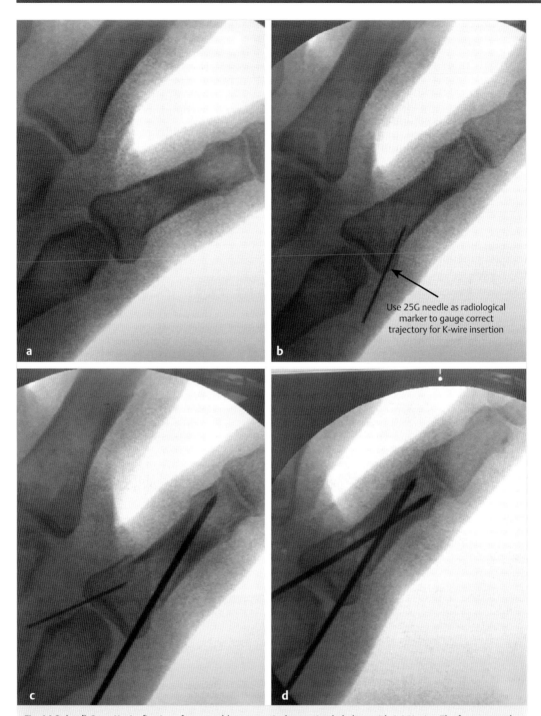

Use 25G needle as radiological marker to gauge correct trajectory for K-wire insertion

Fig. 14.8 (a–d) Cross K-wire fixation of an unstable extra-articular proximal phalanx with 1.1 K-wire. The fracture can be reduced by traction and the flexing of the MCPJ. Note the use of 25-gauge orange needles as radiologic markers. Satisfactory reduction was achieved and rotational deformity was corrected.

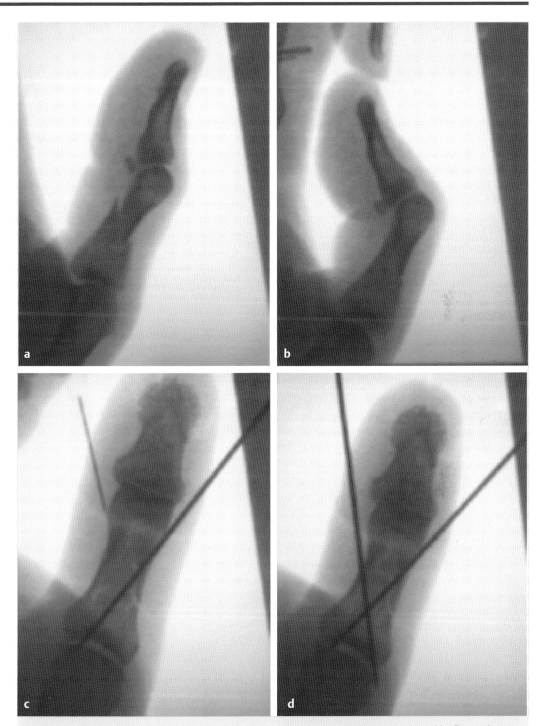

Fig. 14.9 (a–d) Cross K-wire fixation of a thumb proximal phalanx fracture. Reduction is achieved by flexing the IPJ, a single K-wire is then passed to achieve stability followed by a second wire.

14.5 Fracture Dislocations of the Base of the Fourth and Fifth Metacarpals

These injuries can be easily missed and that is why it is essential to always examine three views (anteroposterior [AP], lateral, oblique) in the emergency department (▶ Fig. 14.10a,b). They are inherently unstable and even after reduction under anesthesia the base of the fourth and fifth metacarpal will often re-dislocate even in a well-molded plaster cast.

The best approach is closed reduction and Kirschner wires going into the hamate bone from the fourth and fifth metacarpals (▶ Fig. 14.11). Rarely, it is necessary to open these fractures to achieve reduction.

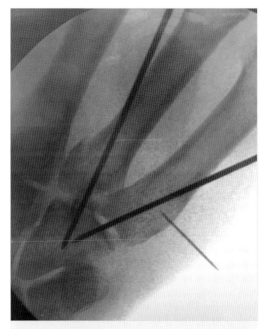

Fig. 14.11 Reduction with two 1.4 K-wires into hamate.

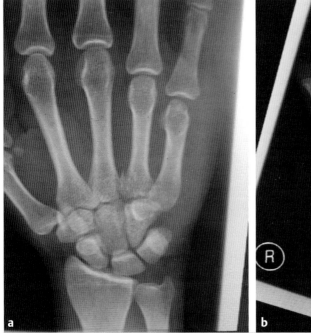

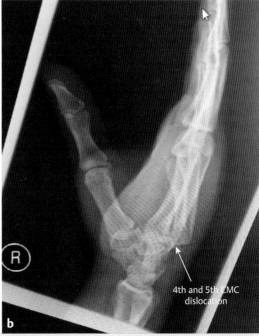

4th and 5th CMC dislocation

Fig. 14.10 With a posteroanterior (PA) view only, fourth and fifth metacarpal fracture dislocation can be easily missed. (a) Lateral view clearly showing fourth and (b) fifth metacarpal dislocation.

14.6 Bouquet Pinning

The case illustrates bouquet osteosynthesis in a neck of fifth metacarpal fracture and a transverse shaft of fourth metacarpal fracture (▶ Fig. 14.12). A 2-cm transverse incision is made at the base of the fourth and fifth metacarpal. The sensory branch of the ulnar nerve is protected and the periosteum off the metacarpal base is lifted off. A burr is used to make a hole of sufficient size to accommodate two or three round-tip K-wires. The Jahss maneuver, as previously described, is performed for reduction before the K-wires are passed into the medullary canal. The bouquet osteosynthesis has the advantage of maintaining reduction without opening the fracture site and interfering with the extensor mechanism. Patients can start early mobilization after this fixation technique.

14.7 Plating of Metacarpal and Phalangeal Fractures

Third and fourth metacarpal fractures can often be managed conservatively unless there is significant displacement or rotation resulting in scissoring. This is because they are supported on either side by the transverse metacarpal ligaments that traverse from the second and fifth metacarpals.

For transverse shaft fractures requiring plate fixation, dynamic compression can be obtained by eccentric screw placement in the plate (▶ Fig. 14.13). The plate is first secured by a neutral screw on one side of the fracture site, then a second screw is eccentrically inserted on the other side of the fracture site. Size 2.0-mm plates should be used for metacarpals, but there are cases when a 1.5-mm plate is appropriate in the smaller adult hand. In the case illustrated, a third metacarpal fracture was fixed with a 2.0-mm plate due to significant scissoring (▶ Fig. 14.14, ▶ Fig. 14.15, ▶ Fig. 14.16, ▶ Fig. 14.17, ▶ Fig. 14.18, ▶ Fig. 14.19, ▶ Fig. 14.20, ▶ Fig. 14.21, ▶ Fig. 14.22).

In some fractures, it is challenging to maintain reduction even with an assistant; a temporary K-wire can be used to hold the fracture before plate fixation (▶ Fig. 14.23). In proximal phalanx fractures, if the fracture configuration is closed, access is through a dorsal curvilinear incision and the extensor tendon is split longitudinally. A

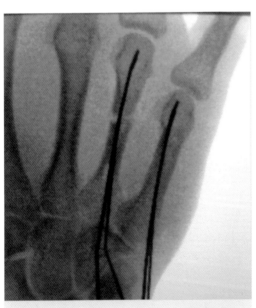

Fig. 14.12 Bouquet osteosynthesis of fourth and fifth metacarpal neck fractures. (This image is provided courtesy of Duncan Bayne.)

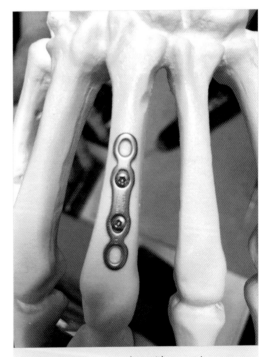

Fig. 14.13 Compression plate with eccentric screw placement.

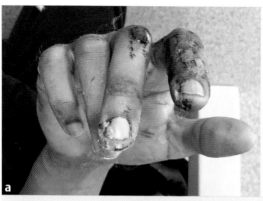
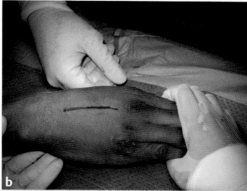

Fig. 14.14 (a) Third metacarpal fracture with significant scissoring. (b) Straight line marking for incision over the third metacarpal in the same patient.

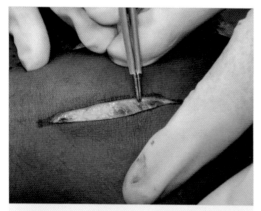

Fig. 14.15 Dorsal veins should be bipolar cauterized. Larger veins need to be tied off with Vicryl.

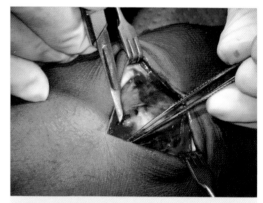

Fig. 14.16 Incision through subcutaneous tissues down to periosteum and hematoma collection. Extensors are pushed to side with retractors.

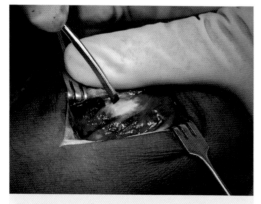

Fig. 14.17 Meticulous preparation of bone ends. Periosteal elevator is used to strip the periosteum off the bone. A Mitchell trimmer can be used to get hematoma and fragments out from the fracture site.

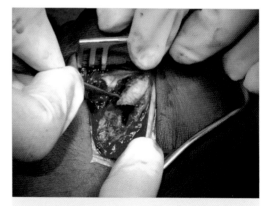

Fig. 14.18 Disimpact the fracture and remove debris with Mitchell's trimmer.

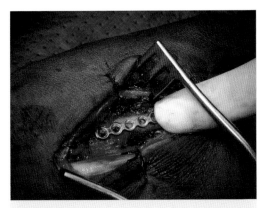

Fig. 14.19 Apply a 2.0-mm plate and use ink to mark the drill sites.

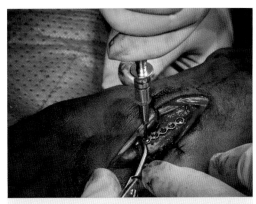

Fig. 14.20 Use a 1.5-mm drill. This provides a better grip for the 2.0-mm size screws being fitted in the figure. Use a depth gauge to ascertain the length of the screw. On some computer X-ray packages, you can also measure out the length of the screw needed.

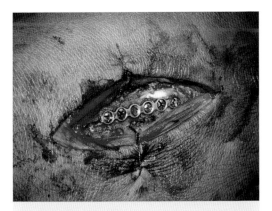

Fig. 14.21 Final result.

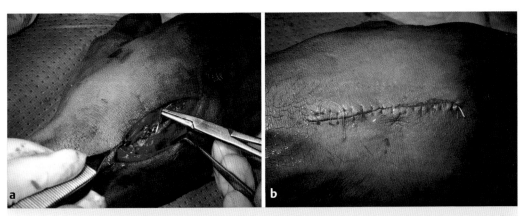

Fig. 14.22 (a,b) Close the soft tissues and what you can see of the periosteum over the plate with 5.0 Monocryl. Finally, close the skin with 5.0 Vicryl Rapide.

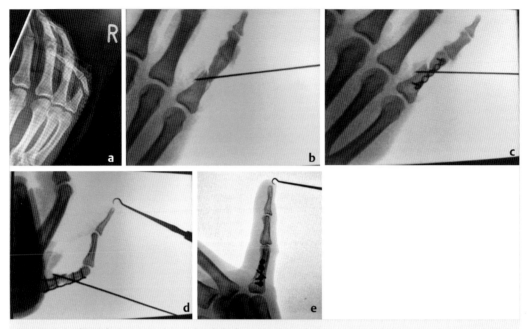

Fig. 14.23 (a–d) Single K-wire can be used to hold fracture in place before proximal phalanx plate fixation with a 1.5-mm plate. (e) Alternatively, the 1.5-mm plate can be placed over the lateral side of the proximal phalanx to avoid problems with the extensor tendon mechanism.

1.5-mm plate can be placed beneath the extensor tendon. An alternative approach is to place the plate over the side of the proximal phalanx to avoid splitting of the tendon and the subsequent risk of tendon adhesions (▶ Fig. 14.23e).

Placing any metalwork in the hand can interfere with tendon glide and these patients should be warned of the possibility of further surgery to remove the metalwork and perform tenolysis.

14.7.1 Rehabilitation of Metacarpal and Proximal Phalanx Fractures

The aim of all internal fixations is to provide a fracture fixation secure enough to allow early mobilization. Open reduction and internal fixation followed by immobilization is a recipe for long-term stiffness.

A forearm-based volar resting splint with the MCPJs in flexion and PIPJs in full extension is used in the immediate postoperative period. This is then changed for a thermoplastic splint. Active motion

exercises are started immediately to prevent scar tethering and reduced motion. Splint protection is also utilized to maintain good joint positions and provide protection as necessary.

14.8 Nonvascularized Bone Grafting

Comminuted fractures with segmental defects require bone graft. The optimal donor site for large defects is from the iliac crest. Smaller defects can be grafted with bone from the distal radius.

A nonvascularized bone graft provides a scaffold for osteoconduction. The case in this chapter illustrates a patient with segmental bone loss after a circular saw injury. A 2×3 cm corticocancellous bone graft was taken from the iliac crest and inset into the first metacarpal with a 2.0-mm bridging plate. If unicortical purchase is taken, a locking plate can be used to provide equivalent strength compared to bicortical fixation (▶ Fig. 14.24, ▶ Fig. 14.25, ▶ Fig. 14.26, ▶ Fig. 14.27).

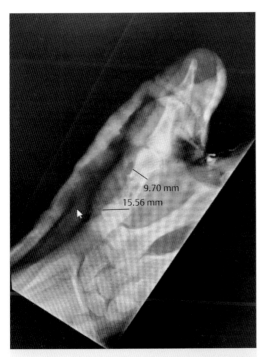

Fig. 14.24 Comminuted first metacarpal fracture with segmental bone loss.

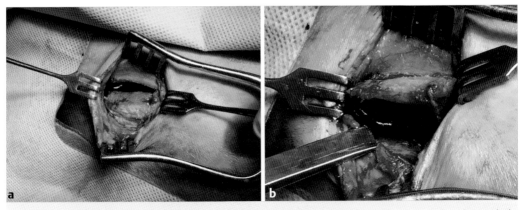

Fig. 14.25 (a,b) Oscillating saw used to harvest bone graft. Osteotome used to lift off bone graft. Defect then packed with bone wax. Care must be taken to avoid the lateral cutaneous femoral nerve.

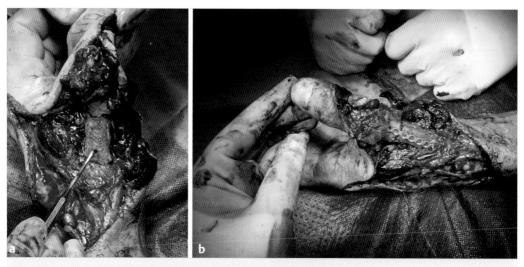

Fig. 14.26 (a,b) Bridging plate placed across nonvascularized bone graft.

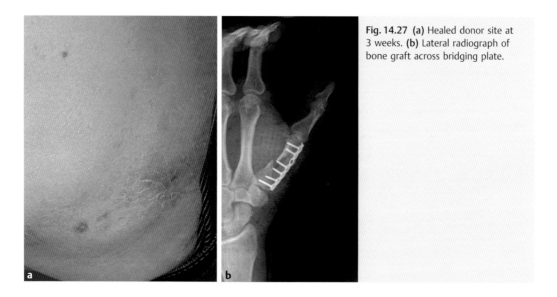

Fig. 14.27 (a) Healed donor site at 3 weeks. (b) Lateral radiograph of bone graft across bridging plate.

14.9 Cerclage Fixation

This is a useful technique to salvage cases where there is significant comminution. Looping interosseous wire through and around fractures can provide some stability. It can be used in combination with K-wire fixation and plate fixation. The case illustrated shows a comminuted middle phalangeal fracture that was stabilized with a cerclage wire and single K-wire. However, it is very difficult to get dental wire around the hypodermic needle. To rectify this problem, we crush the end of the hypodermic needle over the introduced dental wire. This maneuver helps grasp the end of the dental wire, so rather than it being stuck, while being fed through, one can pull the bent needle and thus retrieve the dental wire around the bone. The surgeon can then get two mosquito clamps and grasp each end of the dental wire and tighten it around the fracture (▶ Fig. 14.28, ▶ Fig. 14.29).

14.10 Screw Fixation of Condylar Fractures of Proximal Phalanx

Midaxial access is used to access unicondylar fractures; vertical retinacular fibers are exposed and incised. The extensor mechanism is retracted away and periosteum is incised and cleared away to reveal the fracture line, which is cleaned meticulously. In the case demonstrated, two 1.5-mm screws are passed to fix the fracture (▶ Fig. 14.30, ▶ Fig. 14.31, ▶ Fig. 14.32). If the fracture fragment (▶ Fig. 14.33) is too small to accommodate two screws, a single screw with a 0.9-K-wire cut flush to the bone can be used (▶ Fig. 14.34).

14.10.1 Rehabilitation after Unicondylar Fractures of Proximal Phalanx

The affected digit is splinted ensuring that the IP joints are in full extension. Active motion is commenced early to encourage tendon glide and to prevent an extensor lag of the PIP joint and stiffness.

14.10.2 Screw Size

Screw size includes the width of the thread (▶ Fig. 14.35). Different sets vary but often screw sizes are color coded as in the set shown later. Usually, 2.3- to 2.5-mm screws are suitable for metacarpal fractures, 1.3- to 1.5-mm screws for proximal

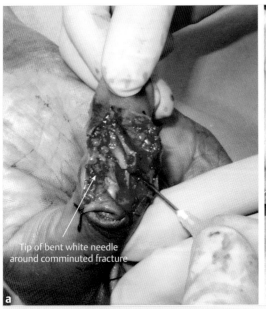

Tip of bent white needle around comminuted fracture

a

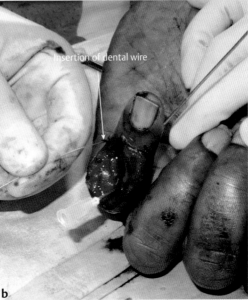

Insertion of dental wire

b

Fig. 14.28 (a,b) Looping around a bent 19-gauge needle to accommodate dental wire for cerclage fixation. The needle must hug the underside of the bone to avoid catching the flexor apparatus and neurovascular bundles.

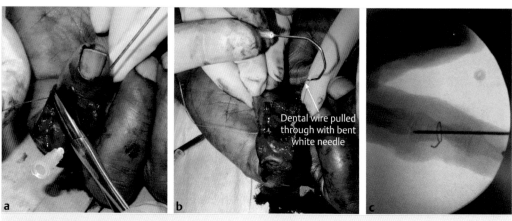

Fig. 14.29 **(a,b)** Dental wire passed through the tip of white needle so that it can traverse around the comminuted middle phalangeal fracture. **(c)** Final radiograph.

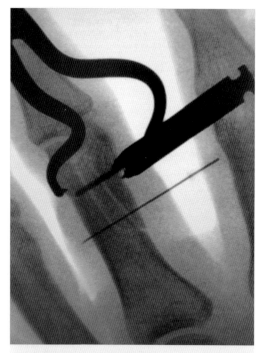

Fig. 14.30 The bicondylar fracture fragments are reduced with a bone clamp and a 1.5-mm screw is passed.

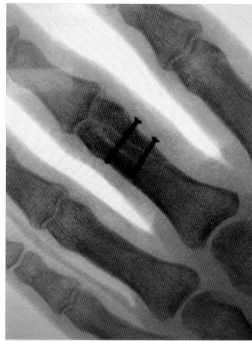

Fig. 14.31 Lag screwing is rarely necessary in hand fractures, and in comminuted fractures such as this it does risk propagating the fracture. Here the fracture has been fixed with two 1.5-mm screws passed through 1.3-mm drill holes.

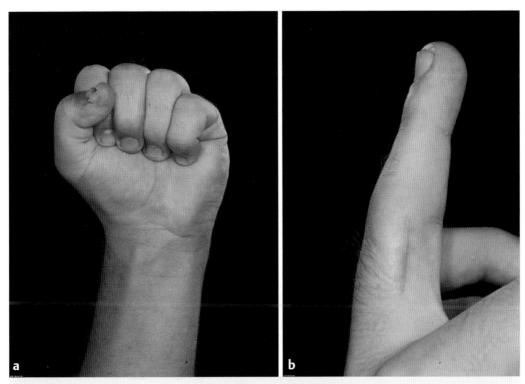

Fig. 14.32 (a,b) Excellent outcome at 3 months in the case in Fig. 14.31 with full range of motion and small scar.

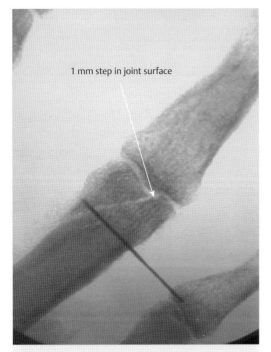

Fig. 14.33 Unicondylar fracture with intra-articular step. Orange needle used to mark placement of screws with ink.

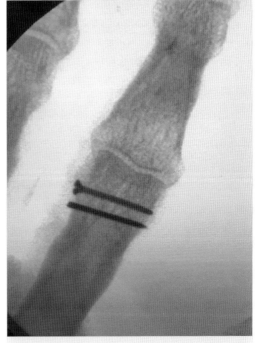

Fig. 14.34 After fixation with 1.5-mm screw and 0.9 K-wire.

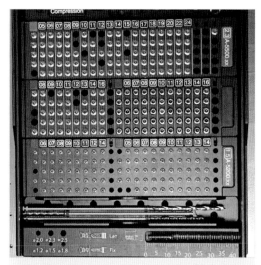

Fig. 14.35 Color-coded fracture fixation set demonstrating variation in screw sizes. Generally, for metacarpals size 2.0- to 2.3-mm plates, for proximal phalangeal fractures 1.3- to 1.5-mm plates, and for middle phalangeal fractures 1.1- to 1.3-mm plates.

phalanx fractures, and 1.1- to 1.3-mm screws for middle phalanx fractures. The color coding system can help identify the correct drill for different-sized screws, but remember, the drill size *must* be smaller than the screw size for the screw to grip.

The exception is lagging when the near cortex is *overdrilled* (or in reality, drilled with a drill that is of the same size as the screw). The lag screw thus does not grip the near cortex (glide hole) but grips the far cortex (which has only been drilled with the small drill). This provides compression. A bicortical interfragmentary screw versus the traditional lag screw is safer and prevents fracture comminution and propagation in small bone fractures.

14.11 Dynamic External Fixation for Pilon-Type Fractures of PIPJ

Pilon fractures are comminuted intra-articular fractures where both dorsal and volar cortical margins are involved and the central articular fragments are impacted into the metaphysis. Secondary to axial loading, there is splaying of bone fragments at the periphery with depression of central articular fragments in the metaphysis.

These fractures are technically difficult to fix once open and therefore dynamic external fixation is a solution. Hynes and Giddins popularized a dynamic external fixator without the use of rubber traction. We detail the steps of frame application using radiologic markers to guide K-wire placement (▶ Fig. 14.36, ▶ Fig. 14.37, ▶ Fig. 14.38, ▶ Fig. 14.39, ▶ Fig. 14.40, ▶ Fig. 14.41, ▶ Fig. 14.42, ▶ Fig. 14.43). Another solution is the pins and rubber traction system described by Suzuki (▶ Fig. 14.44).

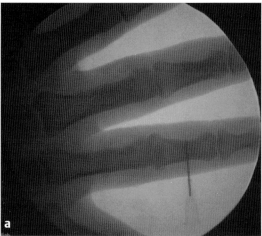
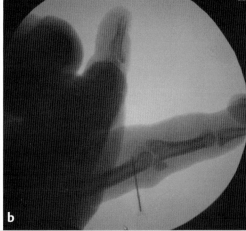

Fig. 14.36 (a,b) Radiologic markers such as 25-gauge orange needles are used to identify proximal and distal K-wire insertion. One can use the needles as cross hairs on the lateral view to guide placement through the head of the proximal phalanx.

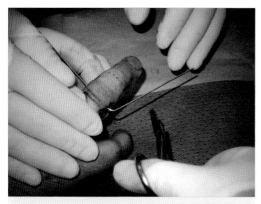

Fig. 14.37 Ink used to mark the head of proximal phalanx and midway through the middle phalanx after the use of radiologic markers.

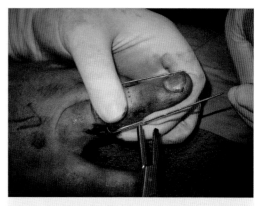

Fig. 14.38 K-wire being centralized so that it does not interfere with rehabilitation. It should be 2 to 3 mm away from the skin edge.

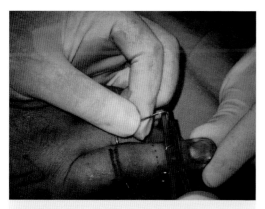

Fig. 14.39 K-wire ends bent into a shape of an S.

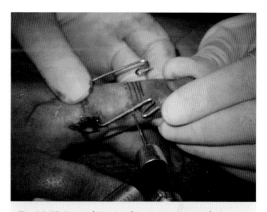

Fig. 14.40 Second K-wire driven approximately 3 to 4 mm proximal to the ink line drawn through the S-shaped hooks of the frame.

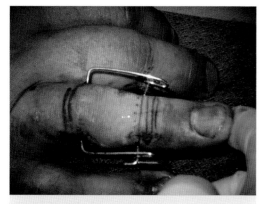

Fig. 14.41 Second K-wire shows some bending suggestive of distraction.

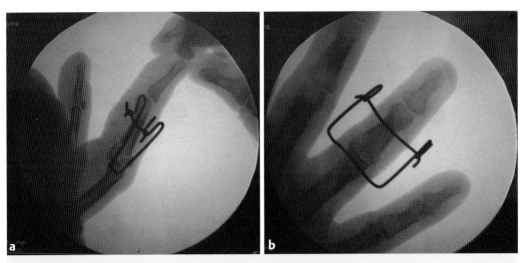

Fig. 14.42 (a,b) Radiographically, distraction is achieved and PA and lateral views are satisfactory.

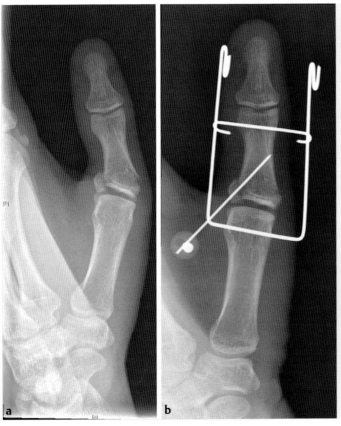

Fig. 14.43 (a,b) Radiographs of Suzuki frame for a pilon-type fracture of the thumb proximal phalanx base.

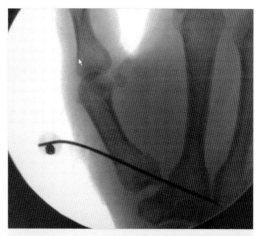

Fig. 14.45 Reduction with single 1.4 Kirschner wire.

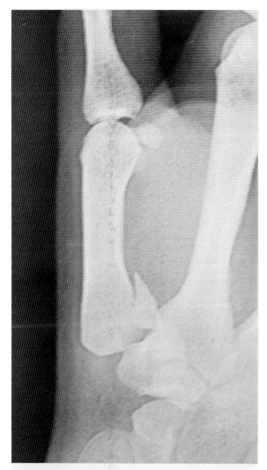

Fig. 14.44 Intra-articular fracture through the base of the first metacarpal.

14.11.1 Rehabilitation after PIPJ Injuries

Loss of PIPJ motion and permanent stiffness are common after these injuries. Therefore, early therapy intervention is essential. Edema control and exercise start on day 3. The dynamic external fixator is usually removed at 3 to 4 weeks.

14.12 Bennett Fracture

This is an intra-articular fracture of the base of the first metacarpal (▶ Fig. 14.45). Reduction is first achieved in these injuries with longitudinal traction and pressure at the thumb base with pronation. A 1.4-size K-wire can then be passed into the trapezium

or base of the second metacarpal (▶ Fig. 14.46). Sometimes it is necessary to pass an additional K-wire for stability into the second metacarpal.

If there is a large bone fragment, a volar approach through the junction of glabrous and nonglabrous skin can be used to gain access and perform lag screw or plate fixation.

14.12.1 Rehabilitation of Bennett Fracture

A forearm-based thumb spica splint often replaces the plaster of Paris cast in the first week. If rigid fixation with a plate is used, active range-of-motion exercises of all joints are started immediately. If K-wire fixation is used, exercises of the IP joint are started at 1 week. The K-wire is removed at 3 to 4 weeks and a splint is worn for protection until fracture healing.

14.13 Bony Mallet Injuries

These are fractures of the distal phalanx where the extensor tendon has come off with a fragment of bone (▶ Fig. 14.47). They often present as closed injuries with extensor lag (▶ Fig. 14.48). In most cases, these injuries should be managed conservatively in a thermoplastic or aluminum splint for 6 weeks (▶ Fig. 14.49, ▶ Fig. 14.50). The patient must not flex the distal interphalangeal joint (DIPJ) during this 6-week period. Splint protection is then worn for the next 2 to 4 weeks.

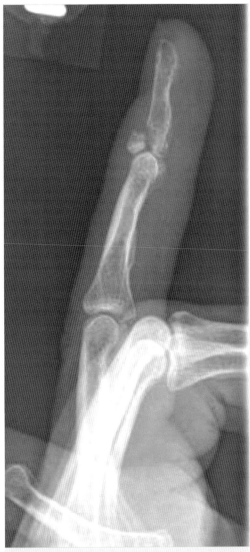

Fig. 14.46 Radiograph of bony mallet fracture without subluxation.

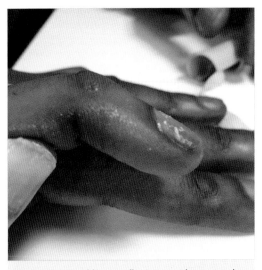

Fig. 14.47 Closed bony mallet injury with extensor lag.

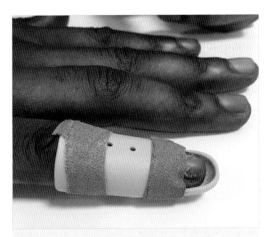

Fig. 14.48 Stack splint. Care to fit these properly as there is a risk of pressure necrosis over the DIPJ.

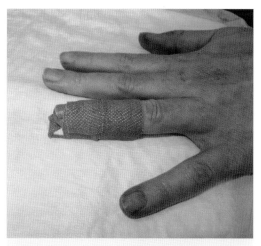

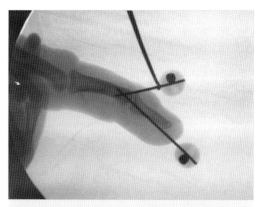

Fig. 14.50 Ishiguro's K-wire fixation of bony mallet.

Fig. 14.49 An alternative method of splinting is with a volar aluminum splint with the DIPJ held in hyperextension.

There are occasions where fixation is needed if the fragments are grossly displaced or if there is subluxation. The subgroup of patients prone to subluxation often have more than one-third fracture surface involved. A lateral hyperextension radiograph as described by Giddins may be helpful in assessing these injuries.

There are many surgical techniques described for fixation. One popular method described by Ishiguro involves a dorsal blocking K-wire passed while the DIPJ is in flexion. The fracture is then reduced and a second K-wire is passed across the DIPJ (▶ Fig. 14.51).

14.14 Static External Fixation

In severely comminuted fractures, it may not be possible to achieve internal fixation (▶ Fig. 14.52, ▶ Fig. 14.53). An external fixator can therefore be applied to bridge the fracture and provide stability. The static external fixator can also be used to stabilize open comminuted fractures that are grossly contaminated. It provides temporary fixation before local or free tissue transfer coverage of a soft-tissue defect.

If an external fixator set is not available, cement passed through a 10-ml Luer lock syringe which has K-wires running through it can be used as in the operative series shown (▶ Fig. 14.54a,b).

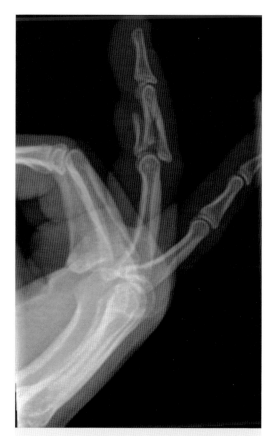

Fig. 14.51 Comminuted pilon fracture of PIPJ.

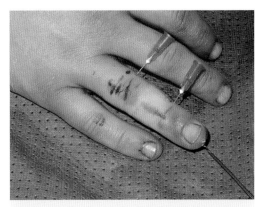

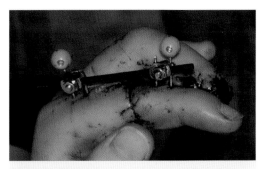

Fig. 14.53 Static external fixator in comminuted P1 fracture.

Fig. 14.52 Radiologic wires to gauge optimal K-wire placement.

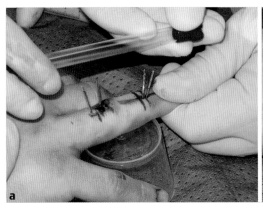

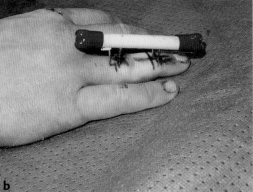

Fig. 14.54 (a,b) Placement of tubing with cement through K-wires for external fixator placement.

Selected Readings

Agarwal AK, Karri V, Pickford MA. Avoiding pitfalls of the pins and rubbers traction technique for fractures of the proximal interphalangeal joint. Ann Plast Surg. 2007; 58(5):489–495

The authors detail their experience with the pins and rubber traction system in a case series of 40 patients. They report unfavorable outcomes and complications and suggest ways of avoiding common pitfalls. The authors emphasized that the traction pin should be centered through the head of the proximal phalanx and the horizontal limb of the traction pin is perpendicular to the long axis of the ray. The vertical limbs of the traction should be appropriately distanced from the digit. A frame that is too wide will interfere with rehabilitation; in contrast, a frame that is too narrow erodes through the skin. Furthermore, true glide should be present during PIPJ flexion so that subluxation does not occur.

Foucher G. "Bouquet" osteosynthesis in metacarpal neck fractures: a series of 66 patients. J Hand Surg Am. 1995; 20(3, Pt 2):S86–S90

The author describes a series of 66 patients that had intramedullary K-wire fixation via an open anterograde technique with prebent round-tipped K-wires. This technique had the advantage of not opening up the fracture site and starting early mobilization. Intraoperative complications in this series included eight incomplete reductions. Postoperative complications included one case of reflex sympathetic dystrophy and one case of dorsal ulnar sensory neuritis.

Giddins GE. Bony mallet finger injuries: assessment of stability with extension stress testing. J Hand Surg Eur Vol. 2016; 41(7):696–700

Bony mallet fractures with a large fracture fragment may be prone to subluxation. The author tested whether extension stress testing on lateral radiographs predicted subluxation. Three patterns were identified on radiographic testing: gliding, pivoting, and tilting. The authors identified a strong association with pivoting and subluxation and gliding and congruence (p < 0.001). The test had a sensitivity of 89% and specificity of 100%. The author concluded that extension stress testing is a more reliable test for subluxation compared to the size of the fracture fragment.

Giddins GE. The non-operative management of hand fractures. J Hand Surg Eur Vol. 2015; 40(1):33–41

Review article discussing available evidence on nonsurgical management of hand fractures. Surgery is often not necessary in many hand fractures and these can be managed conservatively with splinting and physiotherapy. Open fractures and displaced intra-articular fractures almost always need operative fixation. Randomized controlled trials (RCTs) detailing spiral and transverse metacarpal fractures, boxer's fractures, bony mallet, and thumb collateral injuries are discussed.

Ishiguro T, Itoh Y, Yabe Y, Hashizume N. Extension block with Kirschner wire for fracture dislocation of the distal interphalangeal joint. Tech Hand Up Extrem Surg. 1997; 1(2):95–102

Technical paper detailing surgical management of fracture dislocation of the distal phalanx in 84 patients. The DIP and PIP joints are held in maximum flexion. The extension block pin is introduced into the middle phalanx 1 to 2 mm above the fragment. The distal phalanx is pulled distally, and the palmar base of the distal phalanx is pushed up. The DIP joint is then immobilized with a second K-wire.

Nikkhah D, Ruston J, Toft N. Refinements in dynamic external fixation for optimal fracture distraction in pilon-type fractures of the proximal interphalangeal joint. J Plast Reconstr Aesthet Surg. 2016; 69(8):1153–1155

Technical paper detailing steps in application of a dynamic external fixation frame for pilon-type fractures of the PIPJ. The authors use step-by-step images and detail the advantages of this method over pins and rubber traction system. They highlight steps to avoid under-distraction, which is a common mistake in frame application.

Nikkhah D, Sadr AH, Pickford M. Using radiological markers for Kirschner wire fixation of phalangeal fractures. J Plast Reconstr Aesthet Surg. 2016; 69(1):139–141

Technical paper detailing an effective method of planning K-wire fixation of phalangeal fractures with 25-gauge orange needles. Sufficient planning and 3D understanding of the fracture with radiological markers will minimize unnecessary K-wire passes and thermal damage to bone.

Shewring DJ, Miller AC, Ghandour A. Condylar fractures of the proximal and middle phalanges. J Hand Surg Eur Vol. 2015; 40(1):51–58

Case series of 74 patients with phalangeal condylar fractures; 27 patients with unicondylar fractures were operated on using a midaxial approach. All patients regained full range of movement. The author details the steps with excellent intraoperative photographs.

Sletten IN, Hellund JC, Olsen B, Clementsen S, Kvernmo HD, Nordsletten L. Conservative treatment has comparable outcome with bouquet pinning of little finger metacarpal neck fractures: a multicentre randomized controlled study of 85 patients. J Hand Surg Eur Vol. 2015; 40(1):76–83

This randomized controlled trial compared outcomes between conservative treatment of the fifth metacarpal neck fractures and bouquet pinning. Inclusion criteria were where the palmar angulation exceeded 30 degrees. At 1 year, the authors found no differences in QuickDASH score, finger range of motion, grip strength, or quality of life. There were more complications in the operative group (p = 0.02) and greater sick leave (p < 0.001). However, the nonoperative groups were significantly more unhappy with the appearance of their hand; 8/77 who were unhappy had a medial volar angulation of 43 degrees.

Teoh LC, Tan PL, Tan SH, Cheong EC. Cerclage-wiring-assisted fixation of difficult hand fractures. J Hand Surg [Br]. 2006; 31(6):637–642

Technical paper detailing the management of 17 difficult hand fractures that involved butterfly fragments multiple cortical splits or intra-articular extension. The authors detail an elegant method of cerclage-assisted reduction, thus providing sufficient stability for screw or plate fixation. Outcomes were good; at average follow-up of 44.5 months, 17 fractures united without loss of reduction and active range of motion (AROM) was 247 degrees.

15 Local and Regional Hand Flaps

Dariush Nikkhah, Mo Akhavani

Keywords: hand local flaps, regional flaps

15.1 Atasoy V-Y flap

The length of the digit should be preserved and in many cases one can avoid terminalization of the digit. The V-Y flap described by Atasoy is appropriate for dorsal oblique and transverse amputations of the fingertip. To avoid a minimal advancement, it is important to release fibrous septa and detach the flap from the underlying flexor sheath. Through the following illustrations, it is described how to avoid the V-V flap (▶ Fig. 15.1, ▶ Fig. 15.2, ▶ Fig. 15.3, ▶ Fig. 15.4, ▶ Fig. 15.5, ▶ Fig. 15.6, ▶ Fig. 15.7).

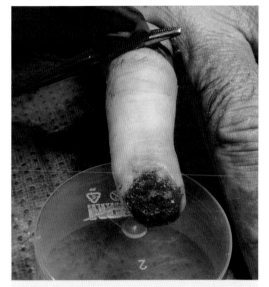

Fig. 15.1 Dorsal oblique amputation of fingertip with exposed bone.

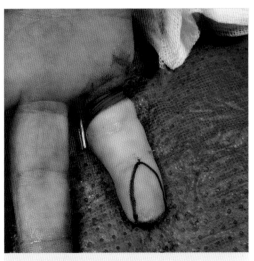

Fig. 15.2 Curvilinear markings, the flap width should be the width of the nailbed.

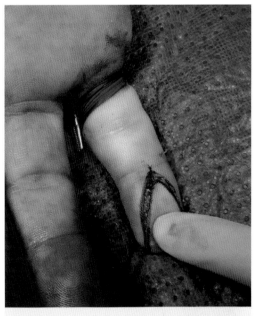

Fig. 15.3 Incision of the skin under digital tourniquet.

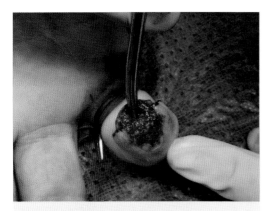

Fig. 15.4 Detachment from flexor sheath.

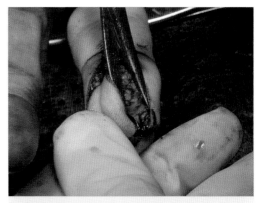

Fig. 15.5 Division of fibrous septa facilitates advancement. The vessels are more elastic in contrast to the fibrous septae.

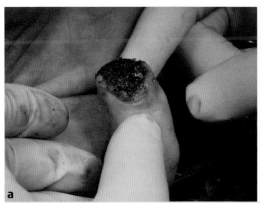

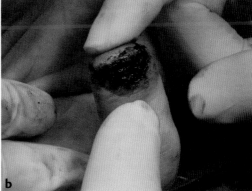

Fig. 15.6 (a,b) Sufficient advancement achieved to provide a well-padded tip.

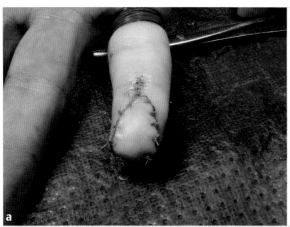

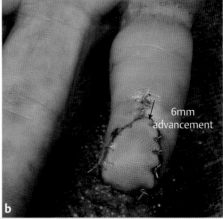

6mm advancement

Fig. 15.7 (a,b) Flap advanced 6 mm, inset with 6.0 Vicryl Rapide, and perfused once digital tourniquet is released.

15.2 Cross Finger Flap

This robust flap is useful in patients who are smokers and have significant comorbidities that could compromise the blood supply of islanded flaps. It is useful for large volar oblique defects of the fingertip and can be divided at 2 weeks. The shortcoming is the poor donor site and ensuing stiffness that can particularly result in adult patients (▶ Fig. 15.8, ▶ Fig. 15.9, ▶ Fig. 15.10).

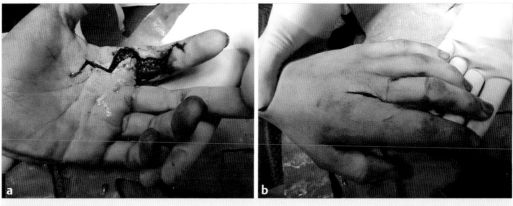

Fig. 15.8 (a,b) Markings for cross finger flap on exposed volar tendon and neurovascular bundle after flexor sheath infection and flap necrosis.

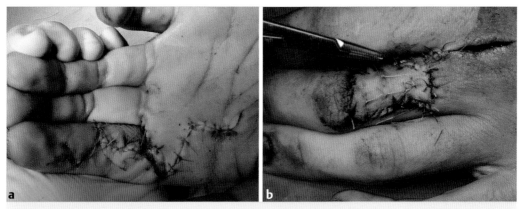

Fig. 15.9 (a) Final result on table with index and middle finger sutured together. **(b)** Donor site full-thickness skin grafted and quilted.

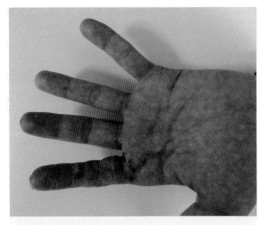

Fig. 15.10 Result at 6 months.

15.3 Venkataswami Flap

This flap is suited to volar oblique defects and involves islanding the flap on its neurovascular pedicle (▶ Fig. 15.11, ▶ Fig. 15.12, ▶ Fig. 15.13, ▶ Fig. 15.14, ▶ Fig. 15.15, ▶ Fig. 15.16). It is often necessary to divide branches from the artery that supply the flexor tendon. For larger defects, more advancement is needed and one must perform the dissection down to the base of the digit.

The Evans flap is a variation which involves creating steps instead of a straight line. This theoretically reduces the chances of scar contracture although it is harder to design.

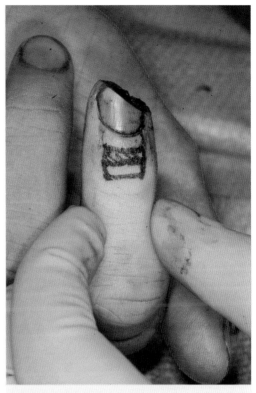

Fig. 15.11 The eponychial flap was not performed in this patient who had an oblique distal tip amputation with bone exposure. Reconstruction with a Venkataswami flap was performed.

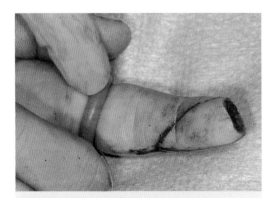

Fig. 15.12 Marking for Venkataswami flap in the same patient.

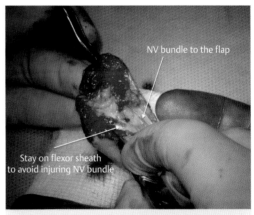

NV bundle to the flap

Stay on flexor sheath to avoid injuring NV bundle

Fig. 15.13 Flap dissection should begin on the side away from the pedicle. The flexor sheath should be hugged and the neurovascular pedicle should be visualized as the flap is being raised away. Incomplete exsanguination of the digit will help in identification of the artery.

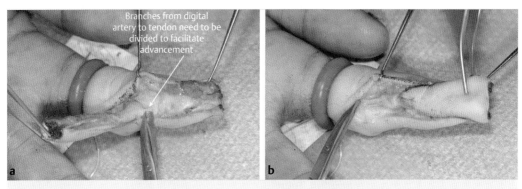

Fig. 15.14 (a,b) Branches from the digital artery to the tendon should be divided to allow advancement.

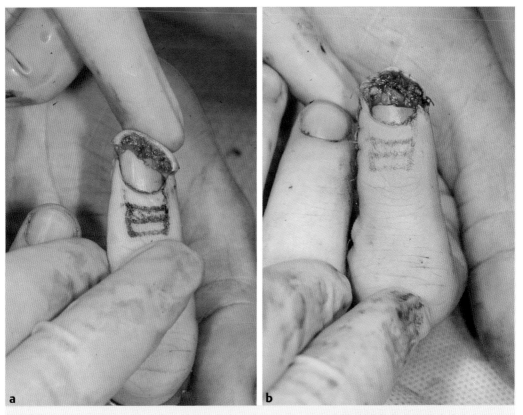

Fig. 15.15 (a,b) Flap advanced nearly 1 cm to provide padded coverage over distal phalanx.

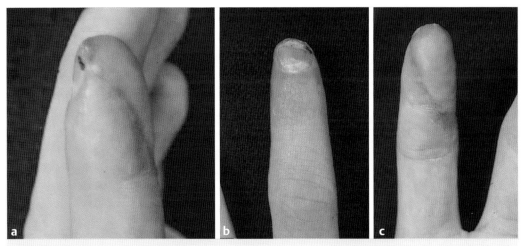

Fig. 15.16 (a–c) Early outcome of reconstruction with normal contour to the fingertip.

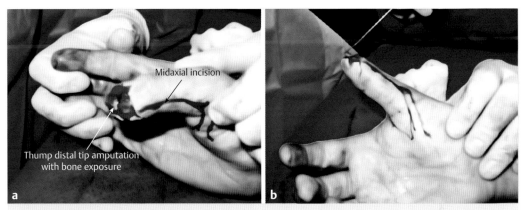

Midaxial incision

Thumb distal tip amputation with bone exposure

Fig. 15.17 (a,b) Skin markings of the Moberg flap. The flap extends to each midaxial line and proximally onto thenar eminence in a V-Y fashion to allow maximum advancement.

15.4 Moberg Flap

Thumb length should be preserved at all costs. To preserve length in volar oblique defects of the thumb tip, a Moberg flap can be performed. This volar advancement flap is raised using two mid-axial incisions and is based on both neurovascular bundles of the thumb, which run closer to the midline than compared to the digits.

In the original description of this flap, the thumb was simply flexed at the interphalangeal joint (IPJ) to gain flap coverage; however, subsequent modifications have involved islanding the flap to gain greater advancement. These include a V-Y plasty over thenar crease (▶ Fig. 15.17, ▶ Fig. 15.18, ▶ Fig. 15.19), or a transverse proximal incision, which is then skin grafted.

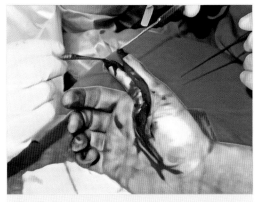

Fig. 15.18 Islanding the volar thumb flap on its two neurovascular pedicles.

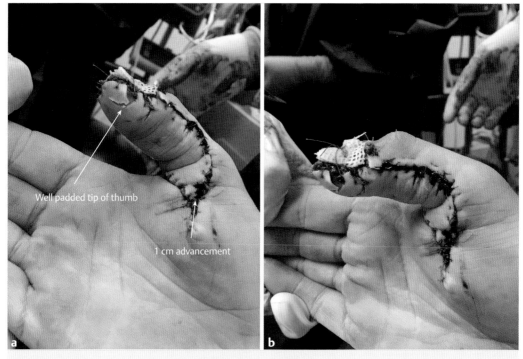

Fig. 15.19 (a,b) Flap advanced 1 cm in V-Y fashion providing sufficient coverage of the thumb pulp.

15.5 The Kite Flap

This flap was originally described by Holevich for thumb reconstruction and later popularized by Foucher. Holevich described a long tail, which protected the first dorsal metacarpal artery from compression. The flap can be used for coverage of dorsal and volar thumb defects and can be neurotized by taking branches of the radial sensory nerve. However, it leaves a poor donor site that requires a full-thickness skin graft (▸ Fig. 15.20, ▸ Fig. 15.21, ▸ Fig. 15.22, ▸ Fig. 15.23, ▸ Fig. 15.24, ▸ Fig. 15.25).

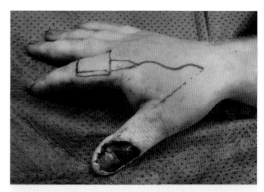

Fig. 15.20 Flap markings for first dorsal metacarpal artery (DMCA) flap for coverage of defect over dorsum of thumb with tendon exposure. The distal margin of the flap should not cross the proximal interphalangeal joint (PIPJ) as this marks the termination of the DMCA.

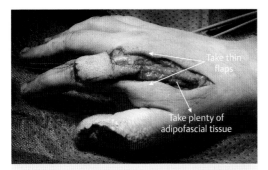

Fig. 15.21 Extremely thin flaps should be raised to preserve the underlying adipofascial tissue, which houses the veins that run alongside the first DMCA.

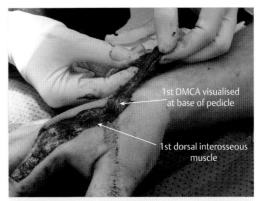

Fig. 15.22 It is not necessary to visualize the first DMCA. Dissection should identify the first dorsal interosseous muscle and all the adipofascial tissues including the fascia over the first dorsal interosseous should be raised.

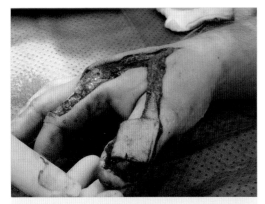

Fig. 15.23 For dorsal defects the flap can be tunneled through, for volar defects it is better to open up the tunnel as passage is longer and traction over the pedicle can result in flap loss.

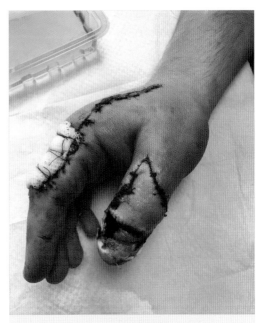

Fig. 15.24 Result at 1 week showing a healthy vascularized flap.

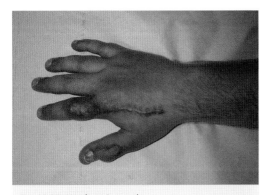

Fig. 15.25 Result at 3 months.

15.6 Retrograde Homodigital Island Flap

This flap is suitable for dorsal and volar fingertip defects. Originally described by Lai, it is designed over a line that corresponds to the dorsal and volar skin. It can incorporate the dorsal branch of the main digital nerve to neurotize the flap. This is particularly important in volar fingertip defects where the restoration of sensation is important,

functionally (► Fig. 15.26, ► Fig. 15.27, ► Fig. 15.28, ► Fig. 15.29).

Several principles which allow ease of execution in this flap include dissection of the digital nerve first and secondly preservation of the adipofascial tissues around the digital artery. The reverse homodigital island flap is reliant on the retrograde blood supply from the arcade around the distal interphalangeal joint (DIPJ). The flap can also be performed antegrade.

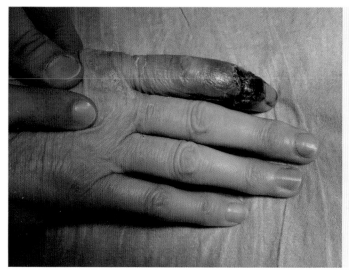

Fig. 15.26 Defect postinfected burn over DIPJ.

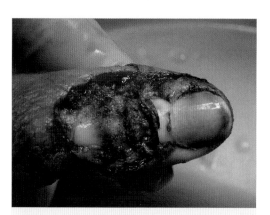

Fig. 15.27 Debridement of tissues and underlying bone.

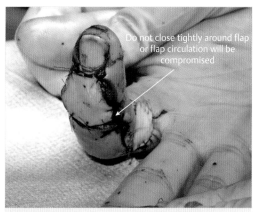

Do not close tightly around flap or flap circulation will be compromised

Fig. 15.28 The homodigital flap is inset loosely. Care must be taken not to tightly close the midlateral incision or the flap will die.

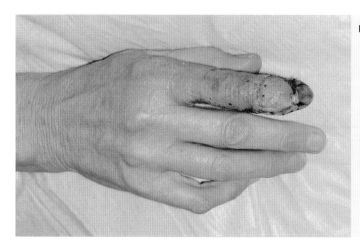

Fig. 15.29 Flap viable at 7 days.

15.7 Reverse Radial Forearm Flap

The radial forearm flap is one of the workhorse flaps in the upper limb. It can be used as a pedicled reverse flow flap for traumatic defects over the hand where tendon and bone are exposed (▶ Fig. 15.30, ▶ Fig. 15.31, ▶ Fig. 15.32, ▶ Fig. 15.33).

A preoperative Allen's test is mandatory to ensure the hand will be adequately perfused by the ulnar artery. Landmarks include a line drawn from the brachial artery to the radial artery, which lies just lateral to the flexor carpi radialis (FCR) tendon palpated near the wrist. The defect is drawn with a template and a length of gauze is used to determine the length of pedicle and pivot point for the flap. Dissection is started laterally over the brachioradialis muscle incorporating the fascia over the muscle and stopping once the septocutaneous vessels supplying the flap are visualized. The cephalic vein is preserved and kept as an additional venous outflow channel for the flap. The lateral antebrachial sensory nerves are preserved, but in some cases may need to be divided. The cut nerve ends are buried in the brachioradialis muscle.

The radial artery is then identified proximally and distally. The radial artery is followed beneath the brachioradialis with the venae comitans,

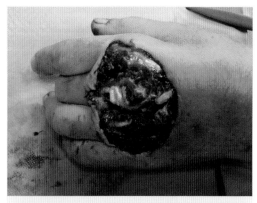

Fig. 15.30 Angle grinder injury resulting in unicortical fracture of the third metacarpal and tendon division of extensor digitorum communis (EDC).

numerous muscular branches are clipped off, but a sufficient adipofascial cuff should be preserved around the pedicle. Care is taken not to divide the superficial branch of the radial nerve. The medial end of the flap is then raised ensuring the perforators that are supplying the flap are preserved. The radial artery is divided proximally ensuring the brachial artery is not divided. The flap is then tunneled across the wrist into the defect.

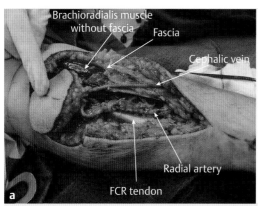
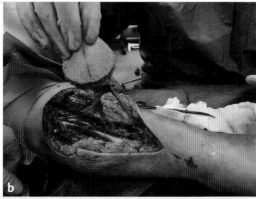

Brachioradialis muscle without fascia
Fascia
Cephalic vein
Radial artery
FCR tendon
a
b

Fig. 15.31 (a,b) Reverse radial forearm flap raised. Note the cephalic vein sitting on the brachioradialis muscle, which is a large fan-shaped muscle. Also, note the pedicle of the flap which has been dissected from underneath the brachioradialis, and in the wrist, it becomes superficial and lateral to the FCR.

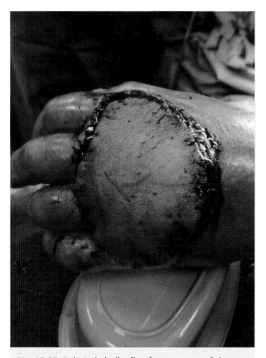

Fig. 15.32 Relatively bulky flap for coverage of dorsum of the hand.

15.8 Posterior Interosseous Artery Flap

This flap does not sacrifice a major vessel in the arm; however, like the radial forearm flap, it has a conspicuous donor site. Its dissection is more complex and there are higher rates of flap necrosis reported in the literature. The posterior interosseous artery (PIA) flap is marked by drawing a line from the lateral epicondyle to the ulnar styloid (▶ Fig. 15.34). The flap outline is then marked with a template of the defect in the middle third of this line. Septocutaneous perforators can be identified by handheld Doppler.

The dissection is started distally identifying the PIA between the extensor digiti minimi (EDM) and extensor carpi ulnaris (ECU) compartment. It is important to take all the adipofascial tissue around the PIA; one can also take a fascial strip over the PIA to protect the pedicle (▶ Fig. 15.35, ▶ Fig. 15.36). Care must be taken not to divide the posterior interosseous nerve. The flap has also been described as a free flap for small digital defects.

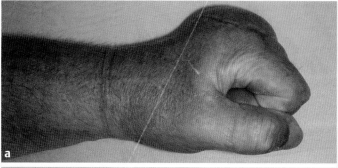

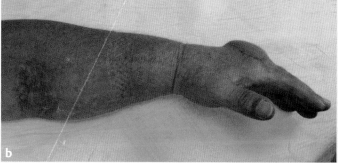

Fig. 15.33 (a,b) Post 6 months, patient achieved full range of motion and opted for no flap debulking.

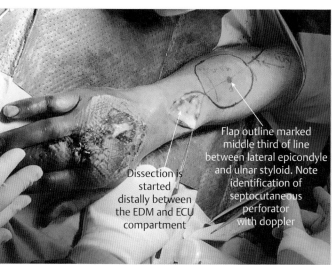

Fig. 15.34 Flap markings with septocutaneous perforator identified with handheld Doppler.

Dissection is started distally between the EDM and ECU compartment

Flap outline marked middle third of line between lateral epicondyle and ulnar styloid. Note identification of septocutaneous perforator with doppler

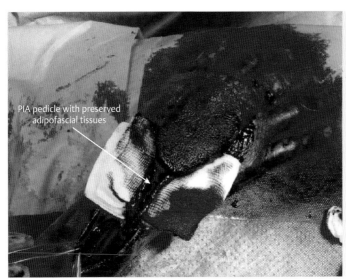

Fig. 15.35 Pedicle taken with wide adipofascial cuff to reduce the chances of congestion.

PIA pedicle with preserved adipofascial tissues

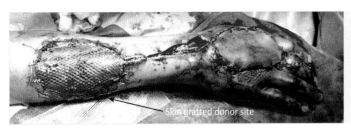

Fig. 15.36 Donor site is grafted and flap inset loosely over defect.

Skin grafted donor site

15.9 Rehabilitation Post Flap Reconstruction

Once the flap is established, early motion of the digits is important. Edema control, scar management to soften and debulk the flap and to improve function are all considered.

Selected Readings

Acharya AM, Bhat AK, Bhaskaranand K. The reverse posterior interosseous artery flap: technical considerations in raising an easier and more reliable flap. J Hand Surg Am. 2012; 37(3):575–582

Case series of 21 patients who underwent PIA flap. All flaps survived without complications. The axis of the flap is the line drawn from the lateral epicondyle of the humerus to the ulnar styloid. The pivot point is 2 cm proximal and radial to the ulnar styloid. The vascular pedicle is located just distal to the junction of the middle and proximal third of the axis line. The Doppler can be used to identify the critical perforator just distal to the midline of the axis. All cases were designed with a tennis racquet–like cutaneous handle. The PIA was identified in the septum between the ECU and EDM.

The authors highlight the importance of taking a wide cuff of adipofascial tissue that houses veins for adequate venous drainage.

Elliot D. Specific flaps for the thumb. Tech Hand Up Extrem Surg. 2004; 8(4):198–211

Review article on different approaches to soft-tissue reconstruction of the thumb. Details of local and distant flaps for reconstruction of the thumb are discussed. Technical diagrams showing tips and tricks to avoid complications and facilitate advancement of local flaps are detailed.

Foucher G, Braun JB. A new island flap transfer from the dorsum of the index to the thumb. Plast Reconstr Surg. 1979; 63(3): 344–349

The authors detail their approach to harvesting a kite flap from the index finger. This is based on the first dorsal interosseous artery and drained by veins in the adipofascial tissues. It can be neurotized by transferring branches with the superficial branch of the radial nerve.

Kaufman MR, Jones NF. The reverse radial forearm flap for soft tissue reconstruction of the wrist and hand. Tech Hand Up Extrem Surg. 2005; 9(1):47–51

The authors review the history, indications, and surgical technique for the reverse radial forearm flap. The authors state that this flap is more versatile than the groin flap, PIA flap, and provides coverage of degloving defects over the dorsum of the wrist, hand, and palm.

Lai CS, Lin SD, Chou CK, Tsai CW. A versatile method for reconstruction of finger defects: reverse digital artery flap. Br J Plast Surg. 1992; 45(6):443–453

The authors detail four types of reverse homodigital island flap (standard, extended, innervated, standard and extended). The article describes technical details on raising this flap and how to neurotize the flap by incorporating the dorsal branch off the proper digital nerve for microneurography. Fifty-two fingers had the reverse digital artery flap for reconstruction in one stage. A two-point discrimination of 3.9 mm was achieved in innervated flaps.

Nikkhah D, Singh M, Teo TC. Avoiding the V-V flap when performing an atasoy V-Y flap. J Hand Surg Am. 2014; 39(10):2122–2123

Technical letter describing maneuvers to facilitate advancement of a V-Y flap in the fingertip. To perform a sufficient division of the fibrous septa, the spreading action of tenotomy scissors can be used to delineate structures. The fine vessels are elastic and relatively robust when responding to stretch and can be readily identified under 2.5 × loupe magnification in comparison to the septa. Once all the septa are divided, significant "give" can be achieved and therefore sufficient advancement. The flap is also elevated and released from the flexor tendon sheath. Sometimes one can allow the donor site to heal by secondary intention; one should avoid closing with multiple sutures as that can compromise the vascular supply to the flap.

Venkataswami R, Subramanian N. Oblique triangular flap: a new method of repair for oblique amputations of the fingertip and thumb. Plast Reconstr Surg. 1980; 66(2):296–300

Technical paper describing a triangular flap based obliquely with the base at the tip of the finger and the apex proximally used to cover an obliquely amputated fingertip or thumb. The technique allows for well-padded, sensitive skin to cover the pulp. By keeping close to the fibrous flexor sheath, damage to the neurovascular bundle is avoided. Sometimes it is necessary to take the dissection down to the base of the digit to allow sufficient advancement of the flap.

16 Free Tissue Transfer

Dariush Nikkhah, Roshan Vijayan, Stamatis Sapzountzis

Keywords: free tissue transfer, anterolateral (ALT) flap, venous flaps

16.1 Free Venous Flap

Venous flap blood supply is from afferent and efferent veins. These flaps have been described for use of small digital defects with flaps being taken from the volar forearm. These flaps are thin, easy to locate, and can be dissected quickly. Furthermore, the donor site morbidity is low.

Free venous flaps can be used when the defect is too large for homodigital or heterodigital flaps. They can also be applied as flow through flaps in cases of revascularization with soft-tissue loss and also as a salvage procedure after unsuccessful local flap coverage.

Venous flaps can either be configured with V-V-V or arterialized A-V-V or flow through A-V-A (Chen's venous flap classification). Higher flow rates such as in arterialized venous flaps have more chance of success.

In the case illustrated, the palmaris longus (PL) was identified and marked. A 2×5 cm skin flap was designed along with two superficial veins, which were visible entering the skin flap. A tourniquet was applied without exsanguination of the limb in order that the veins be dilated and the flap

harvest easier. The skin flap was raised on a suprafascial plane, and the marked veins were dissected in adequate length. At the level of the PL, the dissection was proceeded deeper so that the PL remained attached to the skin flap (▶ Fig. 16.1, ▶ Fig. 16.2, ▶ Fig. 16.3).

On the recipient site, debridement on the dorsum of the left little finger revealed a tissue defect of 4×1.5 cm along with 2.5-cm gap of the central slip of the extensor tendon. The radial digital artery and a dorsal superficial vein over the head of the fifth metacarpal were prepared for anastomosis. 11.0 nylon was used for microsurgical anastomosis. The patient had an excellent outcome (▶ Fig. 16.4, ▶ Fig. 16.5, ▶ Fig. 16.6).

16.2 Free Anterolateral Thigh Flap

The anterolateral thigh (ALT) flap is a workhorse flap in lower limb and upper limb defects. Drawing a line from the anterior superior iliac spine to the superolateral corner of the patella marks the flap axis. The perforators are within a 3-cm radius circle on the midpoint of this line. A handheld Doppler can be used to mark out the perforators.

This flap can be harvested as cutaneous, fasciocutaneous, musculocutaneous, and even flow through flap. In the case shown, a fasciocutaneous

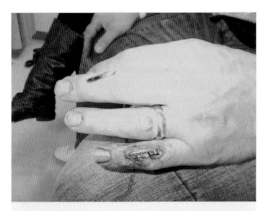

Fig. 16.1 Defect over extensor zone 2 of the little finger with segmental tendon loss and bone exposure 4×1.5 cm defect.

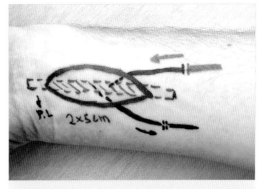

Fig. 16.2 Flap design incorporating PL for dorsal digit defect.

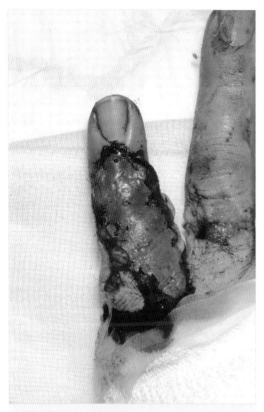

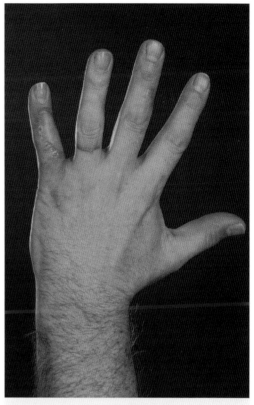

Fig. 16.3 On the third postoperative day, leeches were used for venous congestion.

Fig. 16.4 Full extension achieved.

free ALT flap was harvested for reconstruction of a significant crush defect to the hand.

Flap elevation is started medially; a suprafascial flap can be elevated for a thin flap. In this case, the flap was elevated with underlying fascia. Flap elevation is stopped when perforators are encountered. In 20% of cases, the perforators are identified as septocutaneous and run between the vastus lateralis (VL) and rectus femoris (RF). However, in the remaining 80% of cases musculocutaneous perforators are found traversing the vastus lateralis. A yellow fatty septum between both VL and RF muscles is easily identified distally. It is much easier to identify this septum distally. The RF muscle is displaced medially away from the vastus using a retractor in order to identify the descending branch of the lateral circumflex femoral artery (LCFA) along with its associated perforators. Once adequate perforators are identified, they are traced back to the main pedicle. If the perforators traverse

through the vastus, careful dissection with bipolar cautery can be performed. An alternative approach is "deroofing" the vastus lateralis muscle that lies over the perforators. The tenotomy scissors are slid over the musculocutaneous perforator protecting it while performing cutting monopolar over the vastus muscle. This technique allows for more rapid dissection of the perforators.

Side branches can be ligaclipped if large and if small heat sink, bipolar technique can be used. This involves holding the side branch with DeBakey's forceps and on the side away from the pedicle performing bipolar cautery to seal the vessel. The DeBakey's forceps act as a heat sinking interposition and protect the pedicle from thermal effects of the bipolar. The skin paddle is then finally incised laterally and the flap pedicle is divided from near its origin at the profunda femoris.

After debridement, the recipient site radial artery and vena comitans were prepared for microsurgical anastomosis. It is useful to mark the recipient and donor vessels with blue ink. This helps with alignment before anastomoses and prevents twisting and possible disruption of blood flow. End-to-end anastomosis of the radial artery to the LCFA was performed with 9.0 Ethilon; the LCFV was anastomosed to the vena comitans with a 3.0 venous coupler (► Fig. 16.7, ► Fig. 16.8, ► Fig. 16.9, ► Fig. 16.10, ► Fig. 16.11, ► Fig. 16.12, ► Fig. 16.13, ► Fig. 16.14).

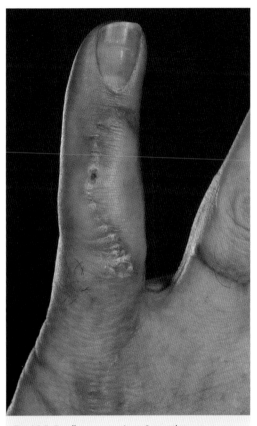

Fig. 16.5 Excellent cosmesis at 6 months.

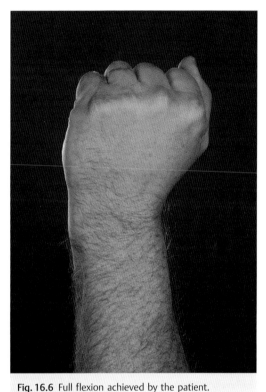

Fig. 16.6 Full flexion achieved by the patient.

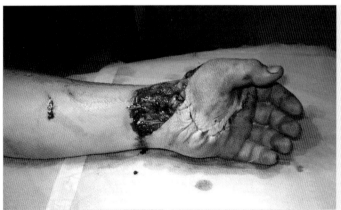

Fig. 16.7 Crush injury to left hand with necrotic tissues beneath degloved skin.

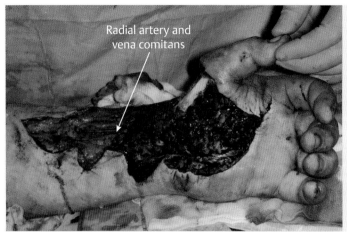

Fig. 16.8 Post meticulous debridement, a large defect with exposed first metacarpal is demonstrated. The radial artery and vena comitans are prepared as recipient vessels.

Radial artery and vena comitans

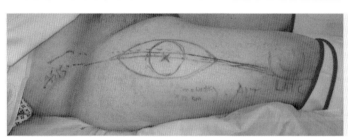

Fig. 16.9 Markings of ALT flap in the same patient with single perforator identified.

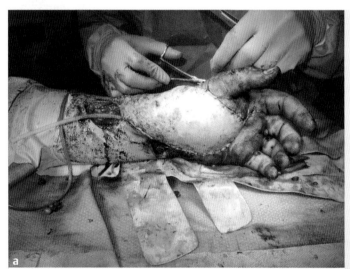

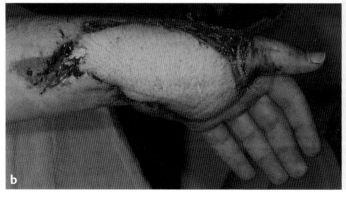

Fig. 16.10 **(a)** Intraoperative inset of flap. **(b)** Flap at 3 weeks.

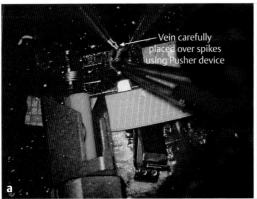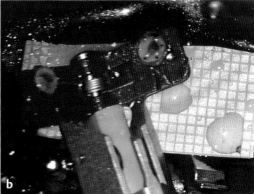

Fig. 16.11 (a,b) Veins anastomosed with venous coupler.

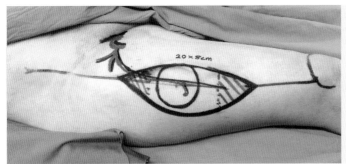

Fig. 16.12 Color markings of ALT flap demonstrating descending branch of LCFA. LCFA, lateral circumflex femoral artery.

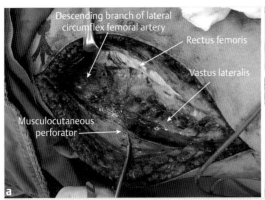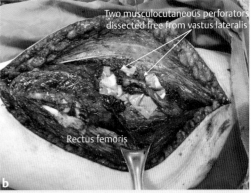

Fig. 16.13 (a,b) ALT flap dissection. Pedicle identified between rectus femoris and vastus lateralis. In this case, two musculocutaneous perforators have been dissected free from the vastus lateralis.

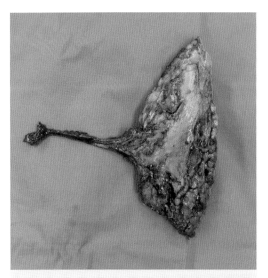

Fig. 16.14 Raised ALT flap demonstrating long pedicle.

16.3 Postoperative Flap Monitoring

Clinical evaluation remains the gold standard for postoperative assessment. A flap should be well perfused with a capillary refill of approximately 2 seconds, skin turgor should be soft, and the flap should be warm. A blue congested flap, with rapid capillary refill is suggestive of venous insufficiency and should be taken back to theater. A pale, cold flap without a Doppler signal is suggestive of arterial failure. Scraping the edge of the flap with a needle to see if there is any bright red bleeding can further assess arterial insufficiency.

Selected Readings

Allan J, Dusseldorp J, Rabey NG, Malata CM, Goltsman D, Phoon AF. Infrared evaluation of the heat-sink bipolar diathermy dissection technique. J Plast Reconstr Aesthet Surg. 2015; 68(8):1145–1151

Animal model examining the thermal effects of bipolar cautery on microvasculature. A comparison was made on a chicken model using the heat sink technique with DeBakey's forceps compared to the standard technique without heat sink. The heat sink model was found to have a highly significant protective effect within 3 mm of important vasculature (p < 0.000000001).

Chen HC, Tang YB, Noordhoff MS. Four types of venous flaps for wound coverage: a clinical appraisal. J Trauma. 1991; 31(9):1286–1293

Article discusses the use of free and pedicled venous flaps to hand wounds in 28 patients. Four types of flaps are described: (1) free venous flaps with total venous perfusion, with ends being anastomosed to two veins, (2) pedicled venous flaps with one end of vein intact and other end anastomosed to a vein, (3) free venous flaps with arterialized venous perfusion with an afferent A-V fistula, (4) venous flaps with total arterialized venous perfusion A-V-A. Arterialized perfusion (type 4) provides the best survival with no flap loss in this subgroup. Small venous flaps were found to survive better than large flaps.

Kayalar M, Kucuk L, Sugun TS, Gurbuz Y, Savran A, Kaplan I. Clinical applications of free arterialized venous flaps. J Plast Reconstr Aesthet Surg. 2014; 67(11):1548–1556

Retrospective case series of 41 flaps. Circulatory abnormalities such as early congestion and edema were seen in 53.6% of cases. A total of four flaps (9.7%) developed necrosis, which presented as full thickness in three flaps and partial thickness in one flap. It can be said that there was a weak but positive correlation between the size of the flap area and the number of anastomosis. The authors also describe the use of syndactylized venous flaps in cases of multiple finger soft-tissue defects.

Wallace CG, Sainsbury DC, Jones ME. A stitch in time, which is perfectly aligned, saves nine. Microsurgery. 2008; 28(5):392–393

Technical paper detailing application of ink microdots over recipient and donor vessels before anastomoses to prevent pedicle malalignment and thus torsion, which could disrupt blood flow to the flap.

Wei FC, Jain V, Celik N, Chen HC, Chuang DC, Lin CH. Have we found an ideal soft-tissue flap? An experience with 672 anterolateral thigh flaps. Plast Reconstr Surg. 2002; 109(7):2219–2226, discussion 2227–2230

This paper details the use of the ALT flap for reconstruction of traumatic and oncologic wounds on various locations in the body. Fifty-eight flaps were used for upper extremity reconstruction. About 87% of the flaps were musculocutaneous flaps. The ALT flap has a long and relatively reliable pedicle; it does not sacrifice any major vessels of lower extremity and has a low donor site morbidity.

17 Limb-Threatening Emergencies

Dariush Nikkhah, Wojtech Konczalik

Keywords: compartment syndrome, escharotomies

17.1 Fasciotomy for Acute Compartment Syndrome

Compartment syndrome is an emergency that if not dealt in time can lead to limb dysfunction and loss. The surgeon should be guided clinically and should not waste time on investigations particularly when signs of compartment syndrome are present. The warm ischemia time for muscle is 6 hours and therefore emergent forearm fasciotomy should be rapidly performed.

The limb in these patients is often tense; there is severe unrelenting pain which cannot be controlled with opiates. Pain is worsened by passive extension. Late signs include diminished pulses.

Surgery involves a long curvilinear incision over the flexor forearm and a straight line incision over dorsal extensor compartment. The carpal tunnel is first released, a U-shaped flap is placed over the wrist and this is to protect the median nerve from exposure. The incision should release the deep and superficial compartments of the arm. The flexor pollicis longus (FPL) compartment is often the most affected. The mobile wad (brachioradialis, extensor carpi radialis brevis [ECRB], and extensor carpi radialis longus [ECRL]) should also be released. Once the patient is stabilized, the wound can be skin grafted with vacuum-assisted closure (VAC). If caught in time, patients can make a full recovery with good long-term outcome (▶ Fig. 17.1, ▶ Fig. 17.2, ▶ Fig. 17.3).

17.2 Hand Compartment Release

This may be necessary in severe crush injuries to the hand: high-pressure injection injuries, reperfusion injuries after replantation, and in circumferential hand burns. The hand has 10 compartments in total and all must be released to prevent muscle necrosis.

The compartments include hypothenar, thenar, adductor pollicis, the four dorsal interosseous muscles, and three volar interosseous muscles. The carpal tunnel must also be released (▶ Fig. 17.4, ▶ Fig. 17.5, ▶ Fig. 17.6, ▶ Fig. 17.7, ▶ Fig. 17.8, ▶ Fig. 17.9).

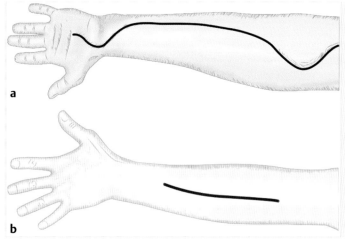

Fig. 17.1 (a,b) Volar and dorsal markings for forearm compartment release.

a

b

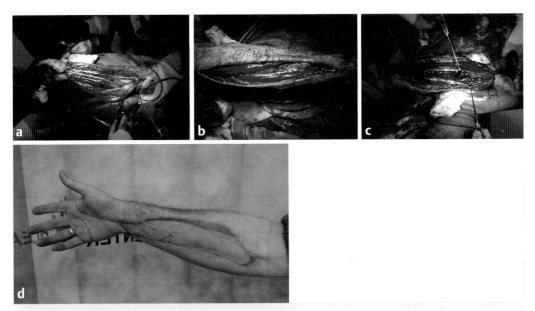

Fig. 17.2 (a–d) Forearm fasciotomies, releasing three compartments in forearm and dorsal compartment with final result and limb salvage in 3 months.

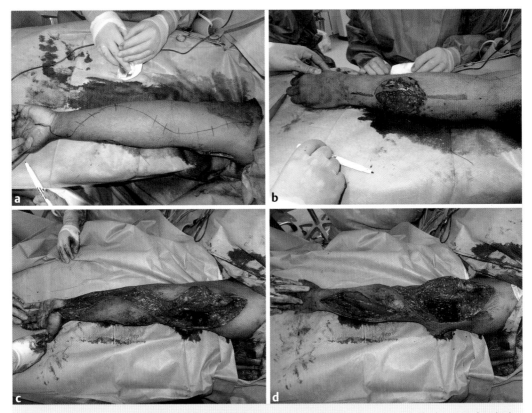

Fig. 17.3 (a,b) Preoperative markings for forearm and upper arm fasciotomies in a patient who had sustained multiple shotgun blast injuries. (c,d) After forearm and upper arm fasciotomy release.

121

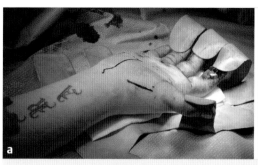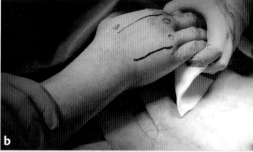

Fig. 17.4 (a,b) Preoperative markings for hand compartment release in patient with crush injury.

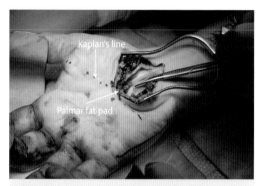

Fig. 17.5 Carpal tunnel release, median nerve contused. Distal extent marked by Kaplan's line and identified by superficial palmar fat pad.

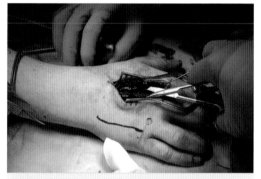

Fig. 17.6 Releasing dorsal and volar interossei through dorsal incisions. Make sure incisions are orientated away from extensors to prevent their exposure.

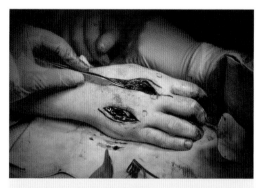

Fig. 17.7 Two longitudinal incisions over the second and fourth metacarpal to release volar/dorsal interossei and adductor compartments.

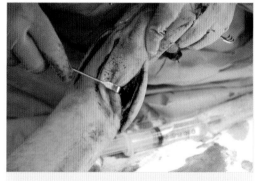

Fig. 17.8 Release hypothenar compartment via incision over ulnar aspect of the fifth metacarpal.

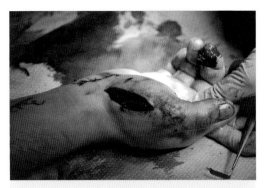

Fig. 17.9 Longitudinal incision over radial aspect of the first metacarpal to decompress thenar compartment.

17.3 Escharotomies

An escharotomy is a technique to treat full-thickness circumferential burns. This enables expansion of the underlying tissues and restores perfusion to the extremity. If there is a failure to restore perfusion, a fasciotomy must be performed.

Upper limb escharotomies are made using a monopolar electrocautery in the midaxial line with the patient's arms in the anatomical position. In the digits escharotomies are best performed using a monopolar with a fine Colorado tip along the midaxial lines. (► Fig. 17.10, ► Fig. 17.11, ► Fig. 17.12, ► Fig. 17.13, ► Fig. 17.14, ► Fig. 17.15, ► Fig. 17.16).

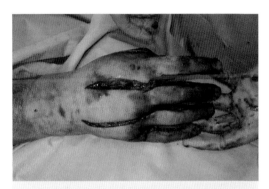

Fig. 17.10 Patient who had sustained a high-voltage electrical injury to both the hands. Decision was made to perform an escharotomy and fasciotomy. In these cases, it is best to use a fine Colorado tip to perform digital escharotomies.

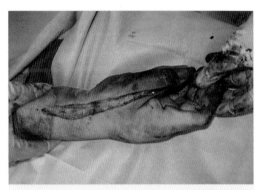

Fig. 17.11 Escharotomy performed on radial side of hand through full-thickness burn into normal tissues.

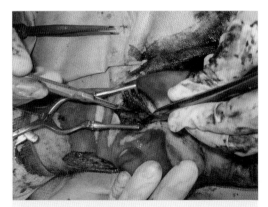

Fig. 17.12 Carpal tunnel release.

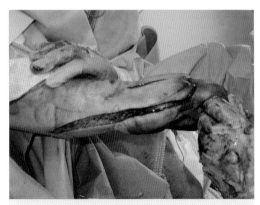

Fig. 17.13 Escharotomy over ulnar side of the wrist and fasciotomy over hypothenar eminence.

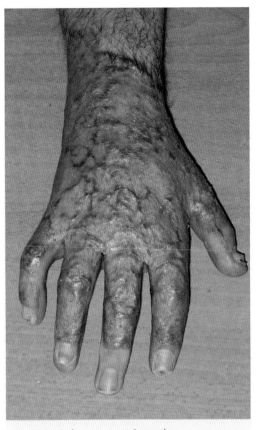

Fig. 17.14 Early outcome at 3 months.

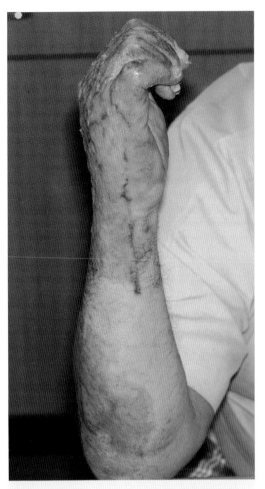

Fig. 17.15 Early outcome at 3 months with limited flexion.

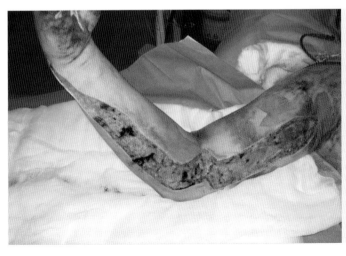

Fig. 17.16 Upper limb escharotomy across midaxial line in a circumferential full-thickness upper limb burn. The incision should extend from unburnt skin to unburnt skin to ensure complete release. (This image is provided courtesy of Baljit Dheansa.)

Selected Readings

Leversedge FJ, Moore TJ, Peterson BC, Seiler JG , III. Compartment syndrome of the upper extremity. J Hand Surg Am. 2011; 36(3): 544–559, quiz 560

Review article on compartment syndrome in the upper limb. The authors discuss relevant anatomy, pathophysiology, treatment recommendation, and outcomes in this challenging condition. Establishing a swift diagnosis is key to avoid limb loss. Acute compartment syndrome involves elevation of interstitial pressures within an osteofascial space. This will in turn result in progressive arteriole collapse and local tissue hypoxia. Early intervention is therefore warranted to prevent cell death.

McQueen MM, Gaston P, Court-Brown CM. Acute compartment syndrome. Who is at risk? J Bone Joint Surg Br. 2000; 82(2): 200–203

Seminal British paper that involved an analysis of 164 patients treated with acute compartment syndrome. Acute forearm compartment syndrome was associated with fractures of distal radius, mainly in young men. Injury to soft tissues without fracture was the second most common cause of the syndrome and was particularly found in patients on anticoagulants. Acute compartment syndrome was diagnosed either clinically or by monitoring of compartment pressure. A differential pressure of less than 30 mm Hg between the tissue pressure and diastolic blood pressure as the threshold for fasciotomy (delta P).

18 Terminalization

Dariush Nikkhah, Amir H. Sadr

Keywords: amputation, terminalization

18.1 Digital Terminalization

There are scenarios where the length of the digit cannot be preserved secondary to either significant trauma, or necrosis due to distal thrombosis of the digital arteries. Terminalization is warranted in these cases to provide a well-padded pain-free stump for the patient.

A fish-mouth incision is designed and the bone is cut back with rongeurs or an oscillating saw to allow for a tensionless closure. Important steps include burying and cauterizing the nerve stumps to prevent neuroma and avoiding the temptation of stitching the flexor and extensor tendons together over the bony stump (▶ Fig. 18.1, ▶ Fig. 18.2, ▶ Fig. 18.3, ▶ Fig. 18.4, ▶ Fig. 18.5, ▶ Fig. 18.6, ▶ Fig. 18.7, ▶ Fig. 18.8, ▶ Fig. 18.9).

18.2 Rehabilitation after Terminalization

Rehabilitation of the terminalized hand/digit and the psychological and functional implications of these injuries should never be underestimated. All patients must be referred for therapy to ensure good motion of the remaining joints, well-shaped stumps with nonsensitive scars; these are all essential to allow patients the chance of an early return to work.

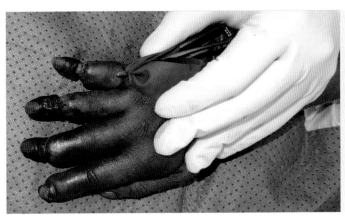

Fig. 18.1 Patient who developed necrotic fingertips after multiple emboli from the subclavian artery.

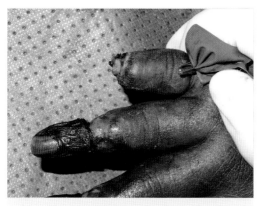

Fig. 18.2 Necrotic segment is removed with a knife demonstrating exposed bone. A digital tourniquet is applied.

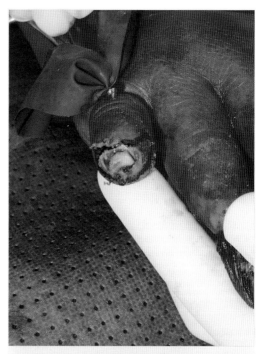

Fig. 18.3 Fish-mouth incision is marked to allow closure of the stump after removal of exposed bone.

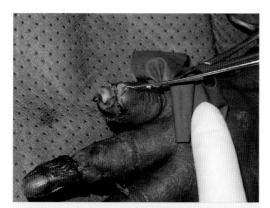

Fig. 18.4 Flaps are raised in a plane just above the bone.

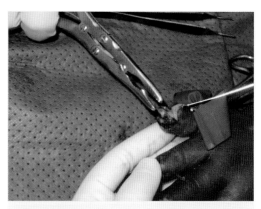

Fig. 18.5 A rongeur is used to remove the bone. If the bone is hard, an electric saw can also be used.

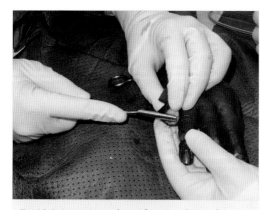

Fig. 18.6 A rasp is used to soften out sharp edges.

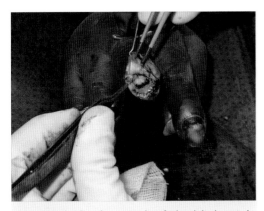

Fig. 18.7 The digital nerve is identified and diathermied using bipolar then cut under tension so that it is buried. The digital arteries are cauterized.

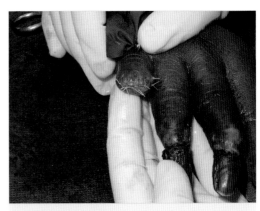

Fig. 18.8 4.0 Vicryl Rapide is used to close the stump, a padded well-protected stump is the result.

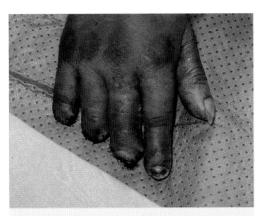

Fig. 18.9 Final result.

Selected Reading

Fisher GT, Boswick JA , Jr. Neuroma formation following digital amputations. J Trauma. 1983; 23(2):136–142

Retrospective study of 144 digital amputations. Only four patients suffered from painful amputation stumps. Only two patients developed neuromas that were resected; the rest of the patients decreased tip sensitivity and they returned to work. The authors felt that the low incidence of neuromas was secondary to patient's desire to return to work early, thereby allowing themselves to do effective exercises to minimize the sensitivity.

Index

Note: Page numbers set **bold** or *italic* indicate headings or figures, respectively.